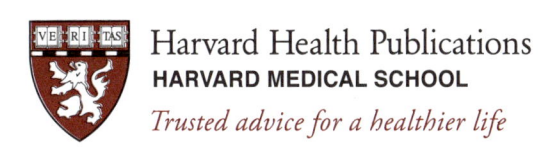

Dear Reader,

Slowly but surely the message is getting out: strength training isn't just for body builders with bulging biceps and rippling abdominal muscles. Like aerobic exercise, it's important for everybody, and everyone should include it in his or her exercise program. Studies show that strength training can help prevent or control conditions as varied as heart disease, diabetes, arthritis, and osteoporosis. This is true whether you're 40 or 85, buff or not. And no matter what your age, it's not too late. The time to start is now, if you want to preserve your quality of life and fight off frailty.

Strength training has many benefits in addition to those listed above. It can tone your muscles and make any sport you play more enjoyable. As you grow older, it can help you perform the tasks of everyday life, such as climbing a flight of stairs, carrying a bag of groceries, or even just putting away a heavy dish in a high cabinet.

Recently we've also begun learning about a related concept called power training, which combines strength training with work on speed. There is overlap between the two, but think of it this way: power training helps you move faster when you walk (allowing you to get across an intersection in a safe amount of time) or react faster (keeping a trip from becoming a fall). The concept of power training was developed in part by my colleagues Jonathan F. Bean and Walter R. Frontera. It was Drs. Bean and Frontera who wrote the original version of this report, which I would like to recognize and acknowledge here.

Muscles naturally weaken with age—starting as early as age 30—so you need to keep working them in order to retain strength and power. The good news is that your investment in exercise can yield quick returns. Studies have found that just 10 weeks of weight workouts can dramatically improve strength, power, mobility, and agility, even in men and women in their 70s and 80s.

In this report, you will find two workouts that include both strength and power training. You'll learn how to begin slowly and safely, and what equipment you need to get started. It isn't much. For our easy-to-follow workouts, all you need are sneakers, comfortable exercise clothes, some small dumbbells, ankle weights, and a sturdy chair. If you already lift weights, you will learn how to step up the pace and keep your routines interesting and fun.

Have fun working out. I know I do!

Sincerely,
Julie K. Silver, M.D.

Medical Editor

The basics: Strength training, power training, and your muscles

Exactly what is strength training? What is power training? How do your muscles respond to these exercises? You'll find answers to these questions below. You'll also learn how muscles work and how aging and disuse contribute to loss of muscle strength and power.

Strength training: The traditional approach

Strength training is a popular term for exercises that build muscle by harnessing resistance—that is, an opposing force that muscles must strain against. Strength training is sometimes called resistance training, progressive resistance training, or weight training. Resistance can be supplied by your body weight, free weights such as dumbbells and weighted cuffs, elasticized bands, or specialized machines. No matter what kind of resistance you use, putting more than the usual amount of load on your muscles makes them stronger. Because the muscles being exercised are attached to underlying bone, these exercises can strengthen your bones as well.

But don't think that strength training is just for twenty-somethings in search of buff bodies or bulked-up muscles. While it can certainly reshape a person's silhouette in a pleasing way, it can also boost the strength everyone needs for daily tasks. Just about any activity becomes easier with stronger muscles. So will any sport you enjoy.

By contrast, weak muscles can make even minor exertion—such as walking a few blocks, climbing stairs, or simply getting out of bed—difficult. Equally important, weak muscles compromise balance. In older people, a debilitating cycle is often set in motion when a fall or disabling condition such as arthritis curtails activity. It's natural to adapt to limitations, but many people find that the less they do, the less they are able to do as time goes on. Fortunately, people can regain their abilities and reverse the cycle with exercises that rebuild lost muscle and help recapture a reasonable range of motion.

Power training: A complementary approach

Another type of training, known as power training, is proving to be just as important as traditional strength training in helping maintain or restore functional abilities.

As the name suggests, power training is aimed at increasing power, which is the product of both strength and speed. Optimal power reflects how quickly you can exert force to produce the desired movement. Thus, faced with a four-lane intersection, you may have enough strength to walk across the street. But can you cross all four lanes of traffic before the light changes? Power, not just strength, can get you from one side to the other safely. Likewise, by helping you react swiftly if you start to trip or lose your balance, power can actually prevent falls.

Some power moves are just strength training exercises done at a faster speed. Other power routines rely on the use of a weighted vest, which is worn while performing certain exercises that are typically aimed at improving functions such as bending, reaching, lifting, and rising from a seated position. But you don't need a vest to do the power training moves we illustrate in Workout I (beginning on page 26).

As you age, muscle power ebbs even more swiftly than strength does. So exercises that can produce gains in power become especially important later in life. That's why some investigators in the field of physical medicine are now combining the swift or high-velocity moves of power training with more deliberate and slow strength training exercises to reap the benefits of both activities.

A look at muscles and movement

Before you read about the health benefits of these forms of exercise or recommendations on which exercises to do, it helps to learn a bit about how your muscles work. Strength training—or actually any voluntary movement in the body—is made possible by skeletal muscles, which are fused to bone. The body boasts more than 600 skeletal muscles. These muscles are composed of many fibers and are surrounded by connective tissue known as the epimysium (see Figure 1, at right). The fibers are grouped together in small bundles known as fasciculi; each bundle is sheathed in connective tissue known as the perimysium.

A muscle seems like a simple thing. But a single muscle may have from 10,000 to over a million muscle fibers (also known as muscle cells). Each of these fibers consists largely of hundreds to thousands of interlocked strands called myofibrils. These, in turn, are built of myofilaments, fundamental muscle proteins that create force. A membrane called the sarcolemma surrounds each muscle fiber and attaches the end of the fiber to a tendon. Tendons are cords of connective tissue that tether muscle to bone.

But a muscle could not contract without nerve impulses. A single nerve cell, or motor neuron, directs activity in a specific group of muscle fibers. Together, this grouping of nerve cell and muscle fibers is called a motor unit. If a given nerve cell commands few muscle fibers, the motor unit marshals less force; the more fibers a nerve cell controls, the greater the force the unit exerts.

When nerve impulses originating in the brain shoot along neural pathways toward a muscle, they trigger a complex set of chemical reactions that cause myofilaments to slide over each other, generating force. Movement occurs when that force ripples through the muscle structure to the tendons, which in turn tug on the bones. Essentially, the bunching muscles act like strings that make a puppet spring to life.

Strength training exercises push muscle beyond its usual capacity. Muscles grow in response to this stimulus because the exercises increase the production of new muscle protein. When this cycle occurs repeatedly, muscles become visibly larger. One theory, tested mostly in animals and a few studies on bodybuilders, suggests that new muscle fibers actually develop in response to microscopic tears in muscle fibers that strength training causes. Interestingly, even if there is no muscle growth, strength training enhances the ability of the nervous system to activate motor units.

Slow-twitch and fast-twitch fibers

Most skeletal muscles have two main types of muscle fibers: slow-twitch and fast-twitch. Usually, a combination of these types gets pressed into service when you exercise. Slow-twitch fibers function best during low-

Figure 1: An in-depth look at muscle

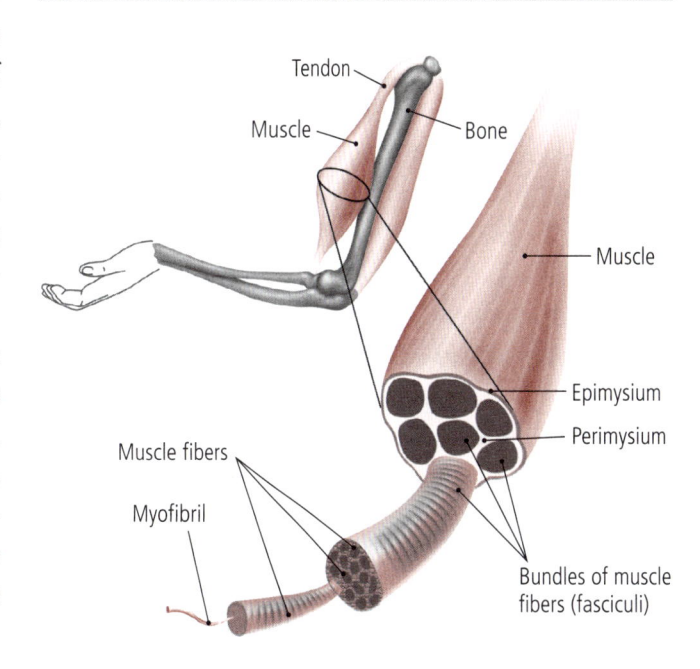

Your muscles are tethered to bone by cords of tissue known as tendons and are covered in connective tissue known as the epimysium. If you could look inside your muscles, you would find that they are composed of small bundles of muscle fibers, known as fasciculi. These bundles are surrounded by connective tissue, or perimysia. One muscle may have anywhere from 10,000 to more than a million muscle fibers. In turn, each muscle fiber consists of hundreds to thousands of tiny, interlocking strands called myofibrils.

intensity activities, when they can be supplied with oxygen. These fibers can keep acting for long periods of time and are called upon first for most activities. During anaerobic activity (a form of exercise that does not require sending significantly more oxygen to the muscles), fast-twitch fibers step into the breach to create bursts of power. Fast-twitch fibers churn out more force than slow-twitch fibers, but are more quickly exhausted. Successful distance runners tend to have greater numbers of slow-twitch fibers in the muscles of their calves, while elite sprinters generally have more fast-twitch fibers. Generally speaking, classic strength training is better for developing slow-twitch fibers, while power training favors the fast-twitch fibers. But in fact, you usually call on both to varying degrees when you exercise.

Studies show that functional activities—that is, activities that people do in their daily lives—also call on both kinds of fibers. Take something as mundane as washing the dishes. The slow-twitch fibers act during most of the slow-paced activity of scrubbing, rinsing, and drying. But when you reach overhead to put away a heavy dish, the fast-twitch fibers get called upon because you are doing something that needs a short but more intense burst of power.

Only a small percentage of muscle fibers available for a task are recruited at one time. More force requires more fibers working in unison. Once they are drained of glycogen (the stored sugar that's their main energy supply), depleted short-twitch and fast-twitch fibers pass the baton to fresh reinforcements so that activity can continue. This relay goes on until you've exhausted the muscle fibers held in reserve.

Muscles at work

Muscles engage in three types of action:

- **Concentric action occurs when muscles shorten and joints move.** An example of this is when you exert the force needed to pick up a bag of groceries.
- **Isometric (static) action creates force, too, but muscles don't shorten or lengthen much and joints do not move.** If you push against a wall, for example, or try to lift an object that is far too heavy for you, you'll feel your arm muscles tense. Since your muscles can't generate enough force to lift the object or shift the wall, they stay in their usual position instead of shortening.
- **Eccentric action occurs when muscles are asked to exert force and move joints while lengthening.** Examples of this would be when you slowly lower a hand weight or walk downhill.

Concentric and eccentric muscle actions are dynamic—that is, they create movement, whether you are jogging or simply walking across a room. Isometric muscle action results in very little movement, such as when a soldier stands at attention or you maintain your balance. Isometric actions are helpful when you want to exercise muscles but have little room to do so or wish to limit movement, such as when joints hurt or are inflamed.

Any time you move, your muscles are applying force. To balance this force properly, different sets of muscles move in opposition to one another. The muscle that delivers most of the force needed for a specific movement—say, walking up a flight of stairs—is called an agonist. To help control the speed and force of the movement and prevent injury, an antagonist that opposes the primary muscle also contracts. So, as you walk up stairs, the quadriceps muscles on the fronts of your thighs act as agonists, while the hamstring muscles at the backs of your thighs work as antagonists.

Age and muscle loss

As the years pass, muscle mass in the body shrinks and strength declines. And it starts earlier than you probably think. Sarcopenia—the gradual decrease in muscle tissue—begins at around age 30. The average 30-year-old can expect to lose about 25% of muscle mass and strength by age 70 and another 25% by age 90.

Some of this muscles loss stems from the physiological effects of aging, but disuse plays a bigger role than many people suspect. Studies of older adults consistently prove that a good deal of the decline can be recouped with strength training.

Similarly, the nerve-signaling system that recruits muscle fibers for tasks deteriorates with age and lack of use. Fast-twitch fibers, which provide bursts of power, are lost at a greater rate than slow-twitch fibers. However, preliminary studies on both power training and strength training suggest that movements designed to restore neural pathways can reverse this effect, too.

It's worth the effort. Having smaller, weaker muscles doesn't just change the way people look or move. Muscle loss affects the body in many ways. Strong muscles pluck oxygen and nutrients from the blood much more efficiently than weak ones. That means any activity requires less effort from the heart and therefore puts less strain on it. Strong muscles are also better at sopping up sugar in the blood and helping the body stay sensitive to insulin (which helps cells extract sugar from the blood). In these ways, strong muscles can help keep blood sugar levels in check—which in turn helps prevent or control type 2 diabetes. Strong muscles enhance weight control, too.

By contrast, weak muscles hasten the loss of independence, putting everyday activities out of reach—activities such as walking, cleaning, shopping, and even dressing. They hinder your ability to cope with and recover from an illness or injury. Disability is 1.5 to 4.6 times higher in older people with sarcopenia than in those with normal muscle strength. Weak muscles also make it harder to balance properly when moving or even standing still—and loss of power compounds the problem. Perhaps it's not surprising that one in every three adults ages 65 and older falls each year. Some of these falls can have dire consequences, including bone fractures, admittance to long-term care facilities, and even death from complications. According to the Centers for Disease Control and Prevention, these spills lead to more than 660,000 hospitalizations a year. But strength and power training can help. People with stronger muscles are less likely to fall and, when they do take a tumble, less likely to sustain a serious injury.

> **Studies of older adults consistently show that much of person's lost muscle can be recouped with strength training.**

Loss of muscle strength and mass aren't the only factors that contribute to age-related declines in functioning and mobility. Research has identified another potential culprit: fat. The Health, Aging, and Body Composition study (commonly called the Health ABC study) revealed that people who have a greater amount of fat between their muscle fibers might be more likely to experience mobility problems.

The location of the fat is a key factor: the fat normally found in muscle cells (intramuscular fat) can provide fuel for exercising muscles, but fat that accumulates between muscle fibers (intermuscular fat) seems to have negative consequences, contributing to insulin resistance, for example. (To visualize intermuscular fat, think of a marbled piece of beef.) Not surprisingly, the amount of intermuscular fat tends to increase with age, as weight creeps up.

The good news is that intermuscular fat responds well to a good diet and regular exercise. One small study published in the journal *Gerontology* supported the theory that even as an octogenarian, you can reduce the amount of fat infiltration in your muscles. In the study, 13 men and women ages 65 to 83 performed resistance training for 24 weeks, stopped the training for 24 weeks, and then resumed it for 12 weeks. After they suspended their routines in the middle phase of the study, the amount of fat in their muscles increased. When they took up their training again, it decreased, even though there was no change in the size of the muscles. More studies are under way to examine how the extent of fat infiltration in muscles affects function and the progression of certain health problems, such as knee osteoarthritis. ▼

What strength and power training can do for you

You've probably heard it all your life: exercise is good for you. Hundreds of studies have demonstrated the truth of this statement. Regular exercise lowers your risks for serious health problems, such as heart disease, type 2 diabetes, high blood pressure, and certain forms of cancer. What's more, it preserves independence, while trimming your silhouette pleasingly. While most studies have focused on aerobic activity, a growing number of strength and power training studies have proven that these forms of exercise deliver significant health benefits as well (see "Benefits at a glance," at right).

This section describes some of the primary health benefits of these forms of exercise, starting with power training, which is newer on the scene and has been studied less extensively.

Health benefits of power training

Football players, high jumpers, and other athletes have long used power training, particularly with weighted vests, to help improve performance.

For non-athletes, there aren't as many studies on power training, but research in this area is growing and has already yielded promising results. The documented benefits include preventing falls, preserving and enhancing physical functioning, and improving quality of life. As this implies, power training in older adults can help stem the progression from gradual impairment to limited daily functioning and then to outright disability. A number of studies have confirmed that power training can make everyday tasks more manageable. In a study in *The Journals of Gerontology: Biological Sciences and Medical Sciences*, researchers reported that while strength training was beneficial, power training was even more effective for improving a person's ability to accomplish daily tasks.

Benefits at a glance

While practically any regular exercise promotes good health, strength and power training can do the following:
- strengthen muscles
- strengthen bones
- prevent falls and fractures by improving balance and preserving power to correct missteps
- ward off loss of independence by keeping muscles strong enough for routine tasks
- help control blood sugar
- relieve some of the load carried by the heart
- improve cholesterol levels
- improve the body's ability to pluck oxygen and nutrients from the bloodstream
- help keep weight within a healthy range
- prevent or ease lower back pain
- relieve arthritis pain and expand a limited range of motion
- raise confidence, brighten mood, and help fight mild to moderate depression.

A 2012 study showed that power training could even help with one daily task that you might not think would improve with exercise—driving. Researchers found that older adults (ages 70 and above) who did 12 weeks of power training leg exercises could brake faster in a driving stimulation than older adults who did 12 weeks of regular strength training exercises or stretching exercises.

There may also be benefits for people with specific conditions. One small study tested three types of exercise—strength training, power training, and stretching—on people with osteoarthritis of the knee. After 12 weeks of exercise, participants in all three groups had better function and less pain, but those in the power training group registered the greatest gains in strength, power, and walking speed. (A second small study found no gains in speed, but did confirm reductions in pain and improvements in tasks of daily living.)

Not surprisingly, these gains can translate into a better quality of life. For a study published in *Health Quality of Life Outcomes*, researchers randomly assigned 45 older adults to a strength training group, a power training group, or a control group that performed no exercise. Both the exercise groups reported improvements in physical functioning compared with those who did no exercise, but only the power training participants reported greater satisfaction with their quality of life.

Health benefits of strength training

Scientists have long known that strength training has a positive impact on your body. Conditions as varied as back pain, heart disease, arthritis, osteoporosis, diabetes, obesity, and insomnia can be partly managed by strength training and other exercise regimens. But what is the relative importance of strength training versus aerobic workouts? Relatively few large, long-term studies have examined this question.

Some things are clear, however. Strong muscles never sleep. Studies have found that strength training can increase your metabolic rate (the rate at which your body converts energy stores into working energy) by up to 15%. This lets you burn more calories, even while you're sitting or sleeping. Coupled with the calories you use up during strength training workouts, this increase in metabolism may help you lose weight or stay at a healthy weight (provided you're eating right).

A solid line of research shows that shaving off as little as 10% of excess weight pays big health dividends. Because obesity factors into many health problems—including high blood pressure, heart disease, gallbladder disease, arthritis, diabetes, and certain cancers—that's an investment that keeps giving back.

Strength training also changes your body composition, gradually replacing fat with muscle. Muscle tissue shrinks with disuse and age. Typically, though, the body doesn't just lose muscle; it replaces muscle with fat. This unkind trade raises the risk for type 2 diabetes, because muscle tissue is better than fat at controlling blood sugar and reducing insulin resistance (the primary cause of type 2 diabetes). In addition, strength training can help peel away an unhealthy girdle of abdominal fat, reducing your risk for heart disease and stroke.

In this section, we have outlined some other ways in which strength training improves specific health conditions, along with tips to consider before you embark on a workout if you have one of these conditions. Here are some of the benefits.

▶ Which is better—strength training or power training?

At the moment, the answer is whichever you will stick with, because studies show that regular strength and power training are both very good for you. One meta-analysis (an analysis of many high-quality studies published on a topic) found that power training had a small advantage over strength training, based on participants' abilities to perform tasks on their own. But finding a program that you'll do regularly is the real key.

Easing arthritis pain

When properly prescribed as part of a larger exercise program, strength training can make a significant difference to people with many types of arthritis.

But arthritis pain presents a difficult dilemma for many people. On one hand, strengthening muscles helps support and protect joints. And exercise, including strength training, helps ease pain, stiffness, and possibly swelling; enhances the range of motion in many joints; and trims excess weight that harms joints. On the other hand, it can be difficult to start weight training if you already have arthritis. Muscles that have not been exercised may be weak and less able to support joints properly. As a result, range of motion, already hobbled by arthritis, is further restricted. But while it may be difficult to strength train initially, doing so typically pays dividends ultimately by improving joint function—provided you begin with light weights or low resistance to avoid joint damage.

Strength training can enhance range of motion in many joints, which is welcome news if you find you no longer have the flexibility to perform basic tasks such as bending down to tie your shoe. In a randomized controlled study of 32 older men, after 16 weeks of workouts, men doing strength training alone or combined with cardiovascular training had significantly more range of motion in seven out of 10 of the joints tested than men who remained inactive. Among those doing just cardiovascular activities, range of motion improved in only two of the joints that were tested.

Strength training can also ease pain and improve quality of life. A study in *The Journal of Rheumatology* found that people with knee osteoarthritis who performed strength training gained strength in their knees, had less pain, functioned better, and reported a better quality of life.

In osteoarthritis, the cartilage that cushions the joints gradually wears away. Another small study suggested that greater quadriceps strength protected against cartilage loss in the knee, since those muscles protect the joint; without strong quadriceps, the joint bears the brunt of the impact, especially when walking or bearing weight. But when the muscles contract, there is a cushioning effect on the joints.

Because excess weight worsens osteoarthritis, strength training's ability to help you control your weight is also important. Adults at a normal weight have roughly a 17% chance of getting arthritis in the knee, compared with adults who are overweight, who have about a 20% risk. Adults who are obese have an even higher risk, at close to 30%. By contrast, according to the CDC, losing even a modest amount of weight can reduce your risk of getting arthritis, or, if you already have the ailment, help reduce pain and improve your quality of life.

People with rheumatoid arthritis can also benefit from strength training, since muscle weakness is common among those with this illness. One study reported that moderate or high-intensity strength training was more effective at increasing or maintaining muscle strength than low-intensity programs. A key to reaping long-term benefits, though, was consistency with the training program. A meta-analysis concluded that strength training not only increases strength, but may also decrease the disability that can result from having rheumatoid arthritis.

"Pre-hab" exercises may deliver benefits after surgery

If you're scheduled to have a joint replacement, don't be surprised if your doctor recommends that you increase your strength and improve your flexibility in the weeks leading up to your surgery. According to studies published in *Arthritis Rheumatology* and in *Physical Medicine and Rehabilitation*, prehabilitation—a combination of resistance training, flexibility exercises, and other exercise done in preparation for joint replacement surgery—may help people who have joints replaced get on their feet faster after surgery, reduce their pain sooner, and show more rapid improvement on the performance of functional tasks.

Tips for people with arthritis

- Have a physiatrist, physical therapist, or certified personal trainer who has experience working with people with arthritis help you design and adapt an exercise program that will work for you. Your exercise program should include strength training, flexibility activities that enhance range of motion, and aerobic activities that avoid further stress on joints, such as water exercise and use of elliptical machines. If necessary, an occupational therapist may be able to suggest splints or assistive devices that will make exercise less painful.
- Schedule workouts for times of the day when your medications are working well, in order to reduce inflammation and pain. For example, avoid morning workouts if stiffness is at its worst then.
- If you have rheumatoid arthritis or another form of inflammatory arthritis, warm-up time that involves gentle stretching is especially important. Inflammation weakens the tendons that tie muscle to bone,

Weight gain and osteoarthritis

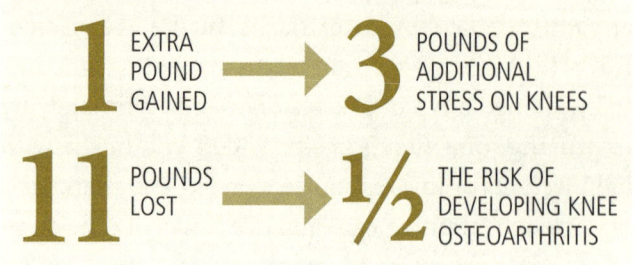

1 EXTRA POUND GAINED → 3 POUNDS OF ADDITIONAL STRESS ON KNEES

11 POUNDS LOST → 1/2 THE RISK OF DEVELOPING KNEE OSTEOARTHRITIS

making them more susceptible to injury. Remember to use slow movements during your warm-up, and gradually extend your range of motion.
- If you have rheumatoid arthritis, strike a careful balance between rest and exercise. When your condition flares up, you will want to rest more to reduce inflammation, pain, and fatigue. When it calms down, you can exercise more. Short rest breaks tend to help more than long periods spent in bed.
- Exercise within a comfortable range of motion, especially while doing upper-body exercises. If an entire exercise causes significant pain, stop doing it! Discuss other options with your trainer or physical therapist.
- Generally, you should avoid doing strength training with actively inflamed joints, at least until the inflammation eases. In some cases, water workouts may be a better choice than strength training.

It's never too late to start

We all want to maintain our health as long as possible. Strength training can slow the downward momentum of old age by rebuilding enough muscle to change life in a host of small yet satisfying ways. Seemingly minor boosts in muscle strength and power in your legs and ankles can reverse snowballing impairments. Some researchers question whether such changes significantly slow or erase disability. Yet small improvements can bridge the gap between rising from a chair unassisted and depending on someone else for help.

That's not the only example. One study found that for some adults 80 and older, 10 weeks of strength training allowed them to forgo a walker in favor of a cane. A study of more than 400 sedentary seniors, ages 70 to 89, found that a yearlong program of strength training in addition to aerobic, flexibility, and balance exercises helped protect mobility. By the end of the study, the participants who exercised were more likely to maintain walking speed for a quarter of a mile than non-exercisers in the control group.

Also promising is a form of exercise known as functional task exercise that helps older adults better accomplish activities of dailing living. Researchers assigned 98 healthy women, ages 70 and older, to one of three groups: a control, a standard strength training program, or a routine designed to more closely mimic everyday tasks. The functional exercises included simple movements, such as carrying a weight quickly across a room or stepping on a raised platform to grab different objects. At the end of the 12-week program, the individuals in the functional exercise group scored higher than the other participants on a test used to measure ability to accomplish daily activities—and the gains lasted six months after training ended. However, the same researchers noted in an earlier study that people who performed both strength and functional routines tended to prefer the strength exercises and were somewhat more likely to stick with them.

Instead of doing a separate functional-task routine, another option is to incorporate an exercise move into your normal day. For example, in one study on people 70 and older who'd had a recent fall, researchers asked one group of subjects to, among other things, do squats instead of bending at the waist to reach for something on a low kitchen shelf. The people doing these functional exercises had fewer falls than those doing strength training exercises; those doing gentle exercises had the most falls of all. (A squat is included in Workout II on page 32. And balance exercises, which help prevent falls, are in both workouts.)

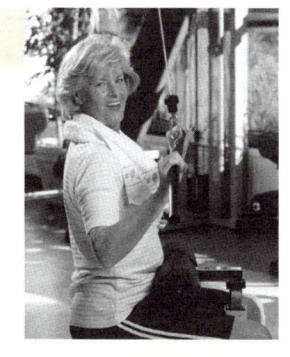

To reap full health benefits, you must increase the weight you use so muscles remain challenged.

The benefits of fitness programs accrue at every age, according to many well-designed studies. That means it's never too late to start an exercise program. Investigators reported in *The Journals of Gerontology: Biological Sciences and Medical Sciences* that after 16 weeks of resistance training, a group of men ages 60 to 75 showed significant gains in strength and muscle fiber size and improvements in aerobic capacity and blood lipids, compared with a control group. Another study comparing strength training, aerobic exercise, and no exercise in healthy women ages 70 to 87 found both the active groups boosted HDL (good) cholesterol and lowered triglycerides (a fat in the blood that, at high levels, is linked to heart disease). Those who did resistance training also lowered their LDL (bad) cholesterol and total cholesterol. While senior programs often focus on very light exercise and stretching regimens, research shows this type of limitation is neither necessary nor especially helpful, as shown in the study described above on functional exercise and falls. Even people hobbled by serious conditions, such as severe frailty or disabling arthritis, can do strength training when other forms of exercise prove impossible. Often, it serves as a gateway to other activities—whether exercise, daily tasks, or purely social pleasures—once a person builds sufficient strength and endurance.

Reducing heart disease risk

Five of the modifiable risk factors for cardiovascular disease—inactivity, high cholesterol, high blood pressure, excess body fat, and diabetes—respond in varying degrees to strength training. Despite this, for years physicians were reluctant to suggest strength training to anyone with a heart condition, fearing it could be dangerous or even fatal. That's no longer the case—at least not across the board. Recommendations from the American Heart Association now suggest that resistance training is safe and beneficial for low-risk cardiac patients, such as people who don't have heart failure, symptoms of angina during exercise testing, or severe heart rhythm abnormalities.

Many cardiologists are willing to extend that exercise prescription further. People who have had heart attacks may start strength training as little as three weeks afterward if their cardiologists recommend it, rather than waiting the more conservative four to six months proposed in older guidelines. In some cases, even some people suffering from heart failure or awaiting heart transplants because of heart failure can benefit from strength training, provided the condition is stable.

A meta-analysis of 12 studies on aerobic exercise, resistance exercise, or a combination of the two in people attending cardiac rehabilitation (where a person might go after a heart attack, stroke, or other serious heart condition) also found that strength training should be part of the picture for people with heart disease. The researchers noted it decreased body fat, increased strength, and improved overall physical fitness as measured by the maximum amount of oxygen a person's body can transport and use during exercise.

By rebuilding muscle, strength training not only gives you more strength for daily tasks, but also helps your body pluck oxygen and nutrients from the bloodstream more efficiently and lightens the load on your heart. If you do strength training regularly, your heart rate and blood pressure are less likely to soar when you perform daily activities like carrying groceries. Such changes may improve heart failure symptoms such as breathlessness and fatigue, too.

There is less information about strength training and stroke (which is sometimes treated as a form of heart disease, because it involves clotting or hemorrhaging in blood vessels that feed the brain). But a 2012 meta-analysis offers some positive news. Though the effect was small, people who did strength training six months after they had a stroke increased both how fast and how far they could comfortably walk.

Tips for people with heart disease

- Talk with your physician before embarking on a strength training program. If your heart disease is mild or well controlled by medications, odds are good that strength training is safe for you. Ask whether you need an exercise test beforehand and a monitored exercise program initially; if so, your doctor may refer you to a hospital, clinic, or cardiac rehabilitation center.
- Strength training is not advised if you have unstable angina, uncontrolled hypertension, uncontrolled heart rhythm disorders, a recent history of heart failure that has not been effectively treated, severe heart valve disease, or hypertrophic cardiomyopathy (a condition in which part of the heart enlarges and obstructs blood flow).
- If you have heart failure, get a baseline exercise test before beginning strength training, and start out in a monitored exercise program. Also, allow 10 to 15 minutes of gentle activity to warm up your muscles, lungs, and heart. Initially, work out at low intensity; interval training—alternating exercise with rest breaks—is fine, if necessary.
- Be sure to breathe while lifting and lowering weights. Holding your breath while straining can raise blood pressure dangerously. Counting out loud as you exhale may help.
- Be aware that many drugs given to help treat heart disease may affect you when you're exercising. Beta blockers, for example, keep heart rate artificially low; that means your pulse is not a good indicator of how vigorously you are exercising. Vasodilators and ACE inhibitors may make you more prone to dizziness from a drop in blood pressure if your post-exercise cool-down is too short. Talk with your doctor about the medications you take. If you work with an exercise professional, be sure he or she understands the potential effects, too.

- If your doctor clears you for strength training, try to choose a supervised program with a certified trainer who understands your condition. Start with a single set (eight to 12 repetitions) of eight to 10 different exercises that target all major muscle groups. Begin with low resistance or light weights. Work at moderate to high intensity: on a scale of 1 to 10, a 5 or 6 would be moderate, while a 7 or 8 would be high. Perform this routine two to three times a week on nonconsecutive days.

Slowing osteoporosis

A combination of age-related changes, inactivity, and poor nutrition conspire to weaken bones over time, with bone mass declining at an average rate of 1% per year after age 40. About 10 million Americans have osteoporosis, which is defined by weak and porous bones, and another 34 million are at risk for it. According to the National Osteoporosis Foundation, about half of all women older than 50, and up to one in four men, will break a bone because of osteoporosis (see Figure 2, at right). This may happen as the result of a fall or even a far less obvious stress, such as bending over to tie a shoelace.

The effects can be devastating. Hip fractures are usually the most serious. One-fifth of seniors who break a hip die within a year from problems related to the broken bone itself or the surgery to repair it. Of those who do survive the hip fracture, many need nursing home care.

Numerous studies have shown that strength training can play a role in slowing bone loss, and several show it can even build bone. This is tremendously useful to help offset age-related decline in bone mass, especially among postmenopausal women. Activities that put stress on bones stimulate extra deposits of calcium and nudge bone-forming cells into action. The tugging and pushing on bone that occur during strength training (and weight-bearing aerobic exercise like walking or running) provide the stress. The result is stronger, denser bones.

Yet strength training has benefits beyond those offered by aerobic weight-bearing exercise. It targets bones of the hips, spine, and wrists, which, along with the ribs, are the sites most likely to fracture. It can help erase another worry, too. Fear of falling can seriously curtail activities of all sorts, especially among older adults. Resistance workouts—particularly those that include moves emphasizing power and balance—enhance strength and stability. That can boost confidence, encourage you to stay active, and reduce fractures by cutting down on falls.

Tips for people with osteoporosis

- Talk with your doctor before beginning strength training. You may need to adapt certain exercises to make them safer. Initially, a monitored workout is best to ensure that you are holding weights safely and using them correctly.
- Research shows that balance exercises significantly reduce falls—more so, in fact, than strength training alone. And fewer falls can mean fewer broken bones,

Figure 2: A fragile state

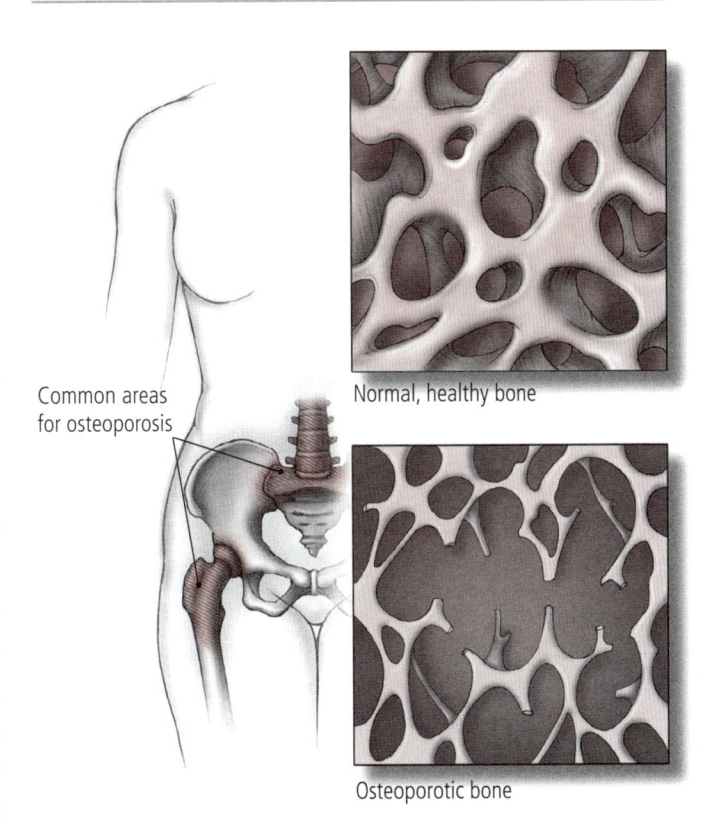

Normal, healthy bone

Common areas for osteoporosis

Osteoporotic bone

Osteoporotic bone is more porous and less dense than healthy bone. The result is bone that is fragile and more vulnerable to breaks. But strength training can slow bone loss and even help build bone.

▶ **A warning for those with joint repairs or replacements**

If any joints in your body have been surgically repaired or replaced, certain exercises may do more harm than good. If you have had a hip repair or replacement, for example, talk with your surgeon before engaging in lower-body strength training. Usually, people are advised not to cross their legs or do any activity that bends the hips farther than a 90-degree angle. You may need to modify certain exercises—such as knee extensions and squats—or substitute different exercises into your routine. Don't write off strength training, though: choosing the right exercises and doing them properly will help strengthen muscles that support the joint.

---

a major cause of temporary or permanent disability. Several of the exercises in this report can help with balance, including the standing calf raise, chair stand, hip extension, and side leg raise. Thigh raises can also improve balance.

- Always choose challenging weights that make it somewhat hard to do eight repetitions, and continue to add weight whenever it becomes easy to do 12 repetitions. The forces associated with muscles contracting and relaxing help to prevent bone loss. (Work with a trainer or physical therapist to help find the right amount of weight that will protect bone without being so heavy that it causes injury.)
- Protect your spine. Strength training exercises that help protect the spine and build strong core muscles include the side bridge (see page 33) and standing side bridge (see page 29). Avoid activities and exercises that require you to bend your spine, especially to lift a weight. This includes bowling, golfing, and even some household tasks. Bend your knees when picking something up. Choose abdominal exercises that lift the head and neck just a few inches rather than bringing your trunk to your knees. Avoid free-weight exercises and machines that put added stress on the spine, such as some leg-press machines, leg raises performed lying down, and squats done with weight bars resting on the shoulders.
- Consider trying exercises using a weighted vest, especially if you are a postmenopausal woman (see "How to use a weighted vest," page 35). Studies have shown that progressive training using a weighted vest can increase the development of new bone in women who have already gone through menopause.
- Because power moves improve your ability to recover your balance quickly and avoid falling, they warrant a place in your exercise routine. For examples, see the standing calf raise, chair stand, stair climbing, and triceps dip on pages 26–28 and "Foot roll: A power move to help you regain your footing," on page 13.

Improving diabetes

If you have diabetes, strength training can help you better control your blood sugar levels. Diabetes is a metabolic disorder characterized by high blood glucose (sugar) levels. It occurs when your body doesn't produce enough insulin (type 1 diabetes) or when your body's cells don't respond properly to insulin (type 2 diabetes). Insulin is a hormone that ushers glucose from the bloodstream into cells, where it supplies energy. If there isn't enough insulin or if the cells don't respond appropriately to insulin, too much sugar remains in the blood, damaging tissues throughout the body.

About 26 million children and adults in the United States have diabetes, and about 11 million of them are older than 65. The vast majority of all people with diabetes have type 2. Strength training and other forms of exercise reduce the risk and impact of type 2 diabetes by improving blood sugar control. Skeletal muscle serves as a reservoir for glucose, penning up blood sugar not immediately needed for fuel in the form of glycogen and doling it out as necessary. Stronger muscles enable the body to more efficiently sop up circulating blood sugar.

Research shows that just one exercise session speeds the rate at which glucose enters the muscles (although that effect dissipates in two to four days unless the activity is repeated). Regular workouts also help the body remain sensitive to insulin rather than succumbing to the creeping insulin resistance so common among older adults. That holds true even if body composition—the percentage of fat versus muscle—stays unchanged.

A meta-analysis looked at 47 studies of people with diabetes who worked out for at least 12 weeks. In these studies, the participants' HbA1c levels, which indicate blood sugar control over the previous two to three months, were lower if they engaged in strength training. This held true whether they did strength training alone or also performed aerobic exercise. Those who did more than 150 minutes of exercise per week saw the greatest declines in blood sugar, as compared with those who did less than 150 minutes per week.

Shaving off pounds by expending calories and boosting metabolism through strength training strikes at another potent risk factor for type 2 diabetes: overweight. A long-term Harvard study published in *The New England Journal of Medicine* traced about 60% of cases of diabetes in 85,000 nurses to excess weight. Strength training has also been shown to reduce the unhealthy girdle of fat that encircles the abdomen. This fat layer, which creates an "apple" body shape (as opposed to a "pear" shape from fat on the hips), is linked to insulin resistance and cardiovascular disease.

When diabetes does develop, strength training can help control it. One study of older adults with type 2 diabetes found that four months of strength training improved blood sugar control so much that seven out of 10 volunteers were able to reduce their dosage of diabetes medicine. This could have particular resonance for blacks, American Indians, and Hispanics, who are more likely than other Americans to struggle with obesity and diabetes.

Even when insulin is not being produced in normal amounts by the body—as is the case with type 1 diabetes—lowering blood sugar through strength training can reduce the amount of injected insulin needed to help keep blood sugar under control.

Tips for people with diabetes
- Talk with your doctor about adjusting your medications before starting a strength training program.
- Take advantage of the fact that strength training is safe and effective for many people who have trouble doing aerobic exercise. That includes frail seniors, some individuals with diabetes, and people with certain disabilities. Check in with your doctor when starting a new exercise program or advancing the one that you are already performing. Your doctor may recommend seeing a physical therapist or physiatrist to help design a workout tailored to your needs.
- Drink sufficient water during and after exercise.
- Wear a diabetes bracelet or ID tag and carry phone numbers in case of emergency while exercising.
- Keep carbohydrates like hard candy or glucose tablets with you when you exercise in case your blood sugar drops precipitously, a condition called hypoglycemia. Signs of hypoglycemia include sweating, trembling, dizziness, hunger, and confusion.
- Lift challenging loads. Blood sugar control has been shown to improve with high-intensity resistance training. Lighter weights or resistance may not have the same effect.
- Consider trying the power move described in "Foot roll," below. One frequent complication of diabetes is deterioration in peripheral nerves, which can diminish sensation in the feet and impair balance. This power move may help you maintain your balance.

Other conditions

Here are a few more ailments that may benefit from regular strength training.

■ **Depression.** A series of studies suggests regular exercise helps lift mild to moderate depression in some people. There is also evidence that people who are physically active are less likely than sedentary folks to suffer from depression in the first place.

Foot roll: A power move to help you regain your footing

People with diabetes can suffer a complication called peripheral neuropathy, which compromises sensation in the feet. This condition can hamper your balance and make it hard to regain your footing after missteps.

Adding a power move called a foot roll to your workout may help you respond swiftly when you lose your balance, according to a small preliminary study published in *Archives of Physical Medicine and Rehabilitation*. Stand with your hands holding on to the back of a chair and your feet together. Quickly roll both feet to their outer edges and back again. Do eight to 12 repetitions.

▶ A potent prescription: Exercise

Medications are well-proven lifelines for millions of people, but some physicians routinely write prescriptions for exercise as well. Conditions such as heart disease, arthritis, osteoporosis, diabetes, and insomnia can be partly managed—and sometimes partly prevented—by strength training and other exercise regimens.

In some cases, regular exercise may make it possible for you to cut back on, or even eliminate, certain medications. In this way, choosing an exercise prescription can sidestep or help squelch potentially unpleasant side effects that typically occur when you need higher dosages of medications or multiple drugs. Of course, before discontinuing any medication or changing the dose, talk with your doctor about the role that exercise can play in your treatment needs.

Strength training also has considerable spillover benefits. While you might choose it for a specific reason—for instance, to help unfreeze joints locked up by arthritis—you may find that your regular workouts help you manage or prevent a host of other health problems. No single pill can make the same boast.

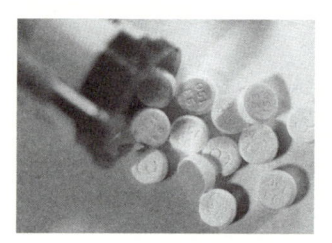

Regular exercise sometimes makes it possible to cut back on certain medications, but talk to your doctor before adjusting your dose.

Thus far, most of the research has focused on aerobic activities, and data from the few available studies on strength training have been mixed. But there are reasons to presume strength training could help. Restoring lost abilities tends to boost confidence and open up new options for pleasurable activities; it may also alleviate dependence on others and fear of falling. Social opportunities offered by exercise programs could provide a lift, as well.

Therefore, strength training mixed with aerobic workouts may be worth a try in combating mild to moderate depression. One study of 60 older adults with depression found that high-intensity strength training was more effective at reducing depressive symptoms than low-intensity strength training, so choose challenging weights and keep working out regularly. Combining exercise with therapy or with both therapy and medication may prove more successful than exercise alone.

See a doctor or mental health professional if symptoms weigh heavily on you or interfere with daily life. Symptoms of depression include changes in appetite; insomnia or oversleeping; feelings of exhaustion, worthlessness, or inappropriate guilt; and agitation or unusual slowness in thinking, talking, or performing tasks. Suicidal thoughts are reason to seek help immediately.

■ **Parkinson's disease.** Preliminary research points to strength training's possible role in managing the debilitating effects of Parkinson's disease. For example, a small study on Parkinson's found that, compared with a control group engaging in other forms of exercise, patients who performed high-intensity resistance training improved their muscle force and walking speed, and boasted higher scores on a quality-of-life questionnaire. Because individuals with Parkinson's often experience slowness in movement, these findings offer hope to them in facilitating activities of daily living.

■ **Down syndrome.** People with Down syndrome typically have significantly less strength than unaffected individuals, according to the American College of Sports Medicine. But one study found that with 10 weeks of strength training exercises, a small group of individuals with Down syndrome improved their upper-body strength by an average of 42% and their lower-body strength by an impressive 90%. Participants also improved their ability to go down steps and get up from a chair.

■ **Lymphedema.** For women suffering from arm swelling after breast cancer surgery, strength training may offer some relief. A study published in *The New England Journal of Medicine* found that of 141 breast cancer survivors who had lymphedema, those who did weight training twice a week for 13 weeks showed an improvement in upper-body strength, reported improvements in their symptoms, and had a lower incidence of flare-ups. In addition, they were no more likely than those in a non-weight-training control group to develop increased limb swelling. These findings call into question the long-held medical view that women who have had breast cancer surgery should avoid stressing the arm for fear that muscle strain could worsen arm swelling. ♥

Getting set up

What you need to get started with strength training depends on the activities you choose. You may opt for a program that relies simply on your body weight, or you might choose to use dumbbells or machines designed for strength training. Some people prefer to work out at a gym or take classes, while others value the flexibility and privacy of a home workout.

With so many products available, you might need some help weighing the pros and cons of each option. Table 1, below, can help you sort through your choices. It describes major categories of strength training equipment and notes their pros and cons.

Buying basic equipment

Want a good home gym you can easily tuck away? This is all you need:

- **Dumbbells in a few different weights.** Depending on your current strength, you might start with as little as a set of 2-pound and 5-pound weights or 5-pound and 8-pound weights. Add heavier weights as needed.
- **Ankle cuffs with pockets** designed to hold weight bars. Brands with 1-pound weight bar inserts are best. Half-pound weight bars may sound easier but make it likely you'll progress much too slowly to make significant gains. When combined, ankle weight bars should add up to about 20 pounds (in other words, 10 pounds per ankle). Depending on the exercises you intend to do, a single ankle cuff may be fine. For the exercises listed in this report, you will need only a single cuff.
- **A nonslip exercise mat** (a thick carpet will do in a pinch).
- **A sturdy chair, preferably with armrests.**
- **A set of weight-lifting gloves (optional).** Gloves work well to cushion hands and keep them from slipping on weights.

Table 1: Choosing strength training equipment

EQUIPMENT	PROS	CONS
Your body weight	• free • always at hand	• can be hard to increase intensity
Elastic bands (also called resistance bands)	• inexpensive • light enough to take anywhere	• difficult to increase intensity • bands become less elastic over time
Free weights (including standard and adjustable weights such as dumbbells or barbells, and ankle or wrist cuffs that hold weight bars)	• fairly inexpensive • good choice at home or at a gym • more muscles and motor units are exercised with free weights, because they are necessary to properly control the weight and achieve good form	• best to have initial supervision or to take a class to ensure good form and safe use; good form is important even if weights are light, but becomes even more so with heavier hand weights and barbells • may be hard to sufficiently increase leg weights in order to progress • as a muscle rotates through a given exercise, its ability to exert force varies at different angles, so the load you lift is limited by the weakest point in your range of motion, and the challenge to the muscle varies
Weight machines (Cybex, Nautilus, Technogym, etc.)	• machine helps ensure good form • easy to add weight as needed • most machines are designed to vary the weight lifted throughout the range of motion of an exercise so that the challenge to the muscle remains optimal • most machines have safety devices	• costly • certain kinds are available only at a gym • best to have initial supervision to ensure you are using the machines safely and properly • momentum may make it easier to lift the load • some machines fail to support or adjust well for women and seniors

- **A weighted vest.** This is optional, but it may be useful for some power moves. When shopping for a vest, make sure to look for one that has pockets for adding or removing weight bars, so you can adjust the weight level to suit your body size and strength (see "How to use a weighted vest," page 35). You can find vests online by searching for "weighted vest," or you may be able to find them at a department store, discount store, or sporting goods store. Prices range from about $50 to more than $200.

Investing wisely in large equipment

If you're considering buying large equipment, choose carefully. The Federal Trade Commission (FTC) warns that quite a bit of the equipment being hawked as part of the multibillion-dollar exercise industry doesn't deliver on its promise. Gather enough information to make a good decision before you spend money.

■ **Avoid equipment or devices that sound too good to be true.** Products that tout easy or effortless muscle gain and weight loss, spot reducing of thighs or waist, and super-speedy results rarely perform as the ads claim they will. The FTC has sued promoters for making exaggerated claims regarding muscle stimulators or abdominal belts that depend on electricity to "exercise" muscles.

■ **Read the fine print.** You may discover that if you want to achieve the promised gains from an exercise machine, you must also follow a low-calorie, high-protein diet high—which can also trim off pounds—or do a surprising amount of exercise.

■ **Be wary of testimonials.** There's no guarantee you'll achieve the same results as satisfied customers, even if the photos aren't airbrushed. Odds are good that any celebrities pictured aren't maintaining their well-toned bodies only by using the equipment they're promoting.

■ **Look at ratings for a range of similar equipment.** Check several fitness and consumer magazines. Articles aimed at people of your age and sex may be especially helpful.

■ **Try out gym machines.** Take free tours of gyms, Y's, and community centers near your home. Ask about the weight machines they have. If one has the kind you are looking for, you might want to take advantage of a one-month or three-month membership. This can be a good test to see whether you would regularly use the equipment or end up hanging clothes on it. Plus, staff members can help you learn to use it safely.

Otherwise, take your time when trying equipment at a showroom or sporting goods store to check for comfort and ease of use. Make sure you understand how to use the equipment properly. Do not buy equip-

Building smarter dumbbells

Dumbbells come in almost as many varieties as ice cream these days. Basic iron dumbbells are generally the cheapest option, although not necessarily the best. Sleek chrome weights look great, but can be hard to hold even when the grip is cross-hatched.

Vinyl-coated, neoprene-coated, or rubber-padded weights are more comfortable to hold and use. Some of these products are color-coded so you can easily pick out the proper weight during workouts.

A nice design in free weights uses threaded metal bars that allow you to attach weight plates at one or both ends. This versatile approach makes it easy to change weights as you gain strength. It also reduces clutter. One good system is the Reebok Speed Pac, which features cushioned grips and removable 2.5-pound weights that can be used in combination to create dumbbells weighing from 2.5 to 25 pounds. Many other systems are also available. Some have less or no center bar padding, but may supply a greater variety of end weights in an easily stowed suitcase.

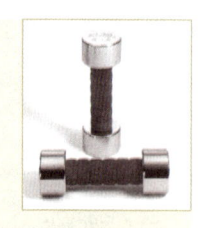

If your hands are arthritic, a padded center bar helps. Or you could consider Reebok's Ironwear hand irons (4- or 6-pound weights) that slip on like fingerless gloves. Other helpful choices include D-shaped coated weights, which are easier to grip, or wrist cuffs with pockets that hold weight bars. Choose styles that feel comfortable to you, such as gel bands or those with padded terrycloth on the inner surface. Wrist cuffs and D-shaped weights may be available only in relatively light weights, however.

You can save money on free weights by buying at a sports resale store. Check your phone book or search online. You might also score a bargain by shopping during annual or holiday sales.

ment that cannot be adjusted to fit your body size. You can also use these strategies if you want to buy a home machine (a treadmill, elliptical, or stationary bike, for example) for the aerobic part of your workout.

■ **Check how easy it is to increase resistance or add weight** in increments of 5 to 10 pounds. Sometimes changing weights is harder than it looks, so try it out. Certain machines can be used with magnetic add-on weights in smaller amounts; ask if that's possible for the machine you're considering.

■ **Look for good construction and safety features.** Strong materials and welds, smooth action, and the right size to fit your space are essential. Cheaper equipment is more likely to be flimsy and unsafe.

■ **Look twice at price.** The FTC warns that "easy installment" payment plans may not include shipping and handling, tax, and set-up costs. Ask exactly what's included. And of course, shop around for the best price.

■ **Consider customer support.** Call toll-free numbers and chat with employees to get an idea of customer support. This is a good time to ask about money-back guarantees and warranties, which may be less enticing if you are responsible for paying to return an item.

■ **Be careful when buying secondhand equipment.** It is cheaper, but warranties aren't likely to apply, and usually you cannot return equipment. If you buy from a gym, the equipment is more likely to be heavy-duty. However, it's also more likely to have seen heavy use.

Personal trainers, physical therapists, and physiatrists

You can certainly follow an exercise program on your own, but exercise professionals can be helpful in certain situations, especially if you want to learn new exercises or are recovering from a health problem.

Perhaps best known are certified personal trainers. These exercise professionals offer one-on-one sessions at a gym or in your home to teach you to work out safely and maintain good form, introduce you to new equipment, and update an exercise program to keep you motivated. They also might push you to work harder than you would on your own.

If you are recovering from certain health problems, you may need to see a physical therapist instead of a personal trainer. Physical therapists help restore abilities to people with health conditions or injuries that affect muscles, joints, bones, or nerves. They create exercise plans that are safe, given a person's injury or medical condition, and they help each client perform the exercise correctly. A physical therapist may specialize in cardiopulmonary rehabilitation, orthopedics, sports medicine, geriatrics, or another area.

Physiatrists are medical doctors who specialize in physical medicine and rehabilitation. Physiatrists treat people who face significant pain, muscle or bone injuries, nerve damage, or conditions such as stroke, hip fracture, or spinal cord injuries that require rehabilitation. Physiatrists may focus on specific areas, such as pediatrics, geriatrics, musculoskeletal medicine, or neurological injuries. While physiatrists may tell you what exercises and movements not to do, they generally leave it up to physical therapists to design exercise programs for their patients.

Insurance coverage varies; in some cases, your insurance may pay for a specific number of sessions with a physical therapist or physiatrist if you are diagnosed with a condition that the company believe warrants the use of such services. Check with your insurance provider to learn more.

Choosing wisely

When selecting an exercise professional, always ask about credentials and experience. Find out how often the person works with people of your age, abilities, and overall health.

In some states, just about anyone can claim to be a personal trainer. Look for someone with certification from the American College of Sports Medicine (ACSM), which offers several levels of training. Another option is certification from the American Council on Exercise (ACE), which offers less rigorous training. You may be able to locate a personal trainer through recommendations from friends or by calling local gyms, Y's, and community or senior centers. Or check with the ACSM or ACE (see "Resources," page 44).

Physical therapists must complete training and pass a national exam given by the Federation of State Boards of Physical Therapy. They should be licensed by

Do I need to join a gym?

No one needs to join a gym to exercise regularly. Your body offers the cheapest equipment available, and spending a little money on other items can deliver great gains. At home, you needn't worry about how you look to others or whether you'll have time to make it to the gym. And the sums saved by not paying for a gym might be put to good use elsewhere, whether that means monthly bills or tennis lessons.

But that doesn't mean that joining a gym doesn't have its benefits. While gym memberships can be costly, spending that money may be an incentive to use the gym regularly and get your money's worth. Classes offer companionship and a safe way to learn technique (provided that the classes are geared toward your ability level). Most good gyms offer a wide range of equipment, so you can try out a variety of strength training machines and exercises. New equipment and a changing roster of exercise classes can keep you challenged and interested in working out. Often, personal trainers are available for weekly appointments or short-term overhauls of your routine. And some gyms offer a post-workout sauna, steam room, or whirlpool that can serve as a nice reward.

Before deciding whether a gym is right for you, consider your preferences and needs. Ask yourself some questions: Do you prefer to work out alone or with others? How far must you travel to the gym, and are you likely to make the trek? Do the gym's hours of operation work well for you? A home gym offers greater flexibility—you can exercise at midnight or 5 a.m. if you wish, but consider whether family interruptions might interfere with a regular workout.

If you decide to select a gym, look for the following:

A good match between your goals and the facility. Plush surroundings and a wide range of amenities cost more. Consider what you really will use—classes, trainers, or just equipment—and ignore the rest. Do, however, choose a gym that's well equipped; a variety of strength training machines and exercise classes allows you to mix up your routine and avoid boredom. And having plenty of equipment can mean no wait, or at least a shorter one, when the gym is busy. Also, be sure that the strength training machines fit you and that resistance is easy to adjust. Because most machines are made with men in mind, this is especially important for women. Take advantage of the fact that many commercial gyms will let you try their facilities for a few days or a week before making a commitment. Make sure you would feel comfortable at the gym during the hours you would normally go.

If you have significant health issues—such as disabling arthritis, a hip replacement, or a serious heart condition—a gym at a hospital or rehabilitation center may offer the best workout for you. Many of these facilities have gyms run by well-trained staff. In some cases, you might be eligible to join a study on exercise that pays the full cost of a specific program while offering excellent supervision by well-qualified professionals.

Well-trained staff. Expertise in teaching people to use strength training equipment and free weights is essential. Ask about staff background and training. Certification from the American College of Sports Medicine is a good sign. Ask whether staff members can perform cardiopulmonary resuscitation (CPR) if necessary. Is a defibrillator available, and do staff members know how to use it? Find out if any trainers frequently work with people of your age, level of fitness, and health status. If you regularly take medications, ask if they know how that might affect your ability to work out. Naturally, a friendly, helpful staff is a plus.

Cost that fits your needs. The Y, community centers, storefront gyms, and even local Boys Clubs and Girls Clubs often offer adult memberships at reasonable prices. Some health care plans offer members discounted rates at specific gyms. Working out only during off-peak hours can cut costs. Some facilities also let you choose to forgo certain amenities, such as a whirlpool and sauna, shower room, or certain classes for a discounted rate. Seniors can often find low-cost or free strength training classes through their local council on aging or senior center.

A well-maintained facility. Before signing a contract, check to make sure that the gym keeps its equipment in good working order. Ask current members if machines are frequently out of order and how long it takes for broken equipment to be repaired or replaced. Also, note whether the public spaces and locker rooms appear clean and well kept.

---

the state in which they practice. Those who complete advanced training in specialized areas must take additional exams to become board-certified specialists.

Physiatrists must complete full medical training and an accredited residency program in their field. Some specialize in specific areas. All must pass written and oral exams given by the American Board of Physical Medicine and Rehabilitation.

If you have significant health problems or disabilities, you can benefit greatly from consulting with a professional who understands your condition before you launch a strength training program. Your primary care physician may be able to refer you to the appropriate person, or you can call rehabilitation centers and hospitals in your area to see if they offer helpful exercise programs for people in your situation. ▼

Safety first

Before you start a strength training program, ask your doctor or physical therapist whether you need to start slowly or take any precautions, such as avoiding certain exercises. It is especially important that you talk to your doctor if you have not been active recently, or if you have any injuries or a chronic or unstable health condition, including:
- heart disease (or multiple risk factors for it)
- a respiratory ailment such as asthma
- high blood pressure
- joint or bone disease
- a neurologic illness
- diabetes.

Some conditions, such as unstable angina or an abdominal aortic aneurysm (a weak spot in the wall of a major artery that may rupture), can make strength training unsafe. Other problems—for example, a joint injury or cataract treatment—may make it unsafe temporarily; in that case, wait until your doctor gives you the go-ahead.

Generally speaking, anyone who is healthy or has a well-controlled health problem, such as high blood pressure or diabetes, can safely do strength training. That includes frail older people. But some people will need more supervision or must observe more restrictions than others.

Questions for your doctor

When you ask your doctor whether to observe any restrictions, it's important to explain exactly what sort of program you hope to undertake. Here are three good questions to ask:
- Do I have any health conditions that would be adversely affected by strength training or other types of exercise? (For example, people with poorly controlled high blood pressure generally should avoid isometric exercises, which can raise blood pressure considerably.)

▶ ### Warning signs

Never ignore these signs of distress from your body. Stop exercising and call a doctor for advice if you experience any of the following:
- upper-body discomfort, including chest pain, aching, burning, tightness, or a feeling of uncomfortable fullness
- wheezing or shortness of breath that takes longer than five minutes to go away
- faintness or loss of consciousness
- pain in bones or joints.

These warning signs pertain to any kind of exercise—strength training and aerobic exercise alike.

Ask your doctor
If you have a chronic health condition, such as heart failure, heart arrhythmias, or hypertension, ask your doctor if you should be alert to any additional symptoms, and keep a record of them—whether that's in a note on your smart phone or on a slip of paper you carry in your wallet. This could be lifesaving information.

- Will my medications affect exercise in any way or vice versa? (People taking insulin or medicine to lower blood sugar may need to adjust the dose for exercise, for example.)
- Should I have any limits on the types or intensity of exercises I do? (For example, some people who have had a hip replacement may be told to avoid bringing their knees to their chests.)

When you may need to stop exercising
The National Institute on Aging notes that there are also specific reasons to hold off temporarily on exercise until a doctor advises you that it's safe to resume. These are not specific to strength training; you should not do aerobic exercise either if you have any of the following:
- a hernia
- sores on feet or ankles that aren't healing
- hot, swollen joints

- difficulty walking, or lasting pain, after a fall
- blood clots
- a detached or bleeding retina, cataract surgery or a lens implant, or laser eye surgery
- chest pains
- fever (it is usually safe to start exercising again at lighter intensity once the fever has subsided and you feel better)
- irregular, fast, or fluttery heartbeat.

Tips for avoiding injury

Strength training is quite safe for most people as long as they take certain precautions. In addition to getting advice from your doctor or other health professional, it's wise to follow these guidelines for avoiding injury:

- Always warm up and cool down properly.
- Use proper form to avoid injuries and maximize gains. It's easiest to learn good form through a class or one-on-one sessions with a well-trained exercise professional.
- Breathe out when you are lifting or pushing; breathe in as you slowly release the load or weight. Never hold your breath while straining. This action, called the Valsalva maneuver, can raise your blood pressure considerably and can be risky for people with cardiovascular disease.
- Lift or push and release weights slowly and smoothly, without jerking.
- Don't lock your joints; always leave a slight bend in your knees and elbows when straightening out your legs and arms.
- Bend at the hips, not at the waist, and keep your back straight.
- Build up slowly over time. Don't be so eager to see results that you risk hurting yourself by exercising too long or choosing too much weight. Remember that it's important to rest muscles for at least 48 hours between strength training sessions.
- If you've been sick, give yourself one or two days off after recovering. If you were ill for a while, you may need to use lighter weights or less resistance when you first resume exercising.
- Slow down if the temperature where you exercise is higher than 70° F. When it tops 80° F, try to exercise only during the coolest part of the day. Dress in loose, light clothes. Headache, dizziness, nausea, fainting, cramps, or palpitations are signs of overheating.
- Drink plenty of water throughout the day and whenever you exercise. As people age, their sense of thirst declines. So it's particularly important for older adults to drink lots of water when they exercise (and throughout the day)—even if they don't feel thirsty.
- Soreness is normal for a day or two after strength training sessions, especially when you first start to work out. But you shouldn't feel overly tired or have sore joints or specific muscle injuries.
- Strength training exercises should not cause pain while you are doing them. When moving your arms or legs, stick with a range that feels comfortable. Over time, gradually extend your range of motion through exercise and stretching.
- Don't overexert yourself. Listen to your body and cut back if you aren't able to finish a series of exercises or an exercise session, can't talk while exercising, feel faint after a session, feel tired during the day, or suffer joint aches and pains after a session. ▼

Quiz: Do you need supervision?

Nearly everyone can exercise, and certainly the vast majority of us should. But for some people it's safest to do so with good supervision. This simple test can help you determine whether you can safely exercise without supervision at home or at a gym, or whether it would be best to work with qualified exercise professionals at a gym, senior center, rehabilitation center, or hospital. Classes taught by well-trained exercise professionals could also be an option.

The test focuses on having adequate balance and a minimal amount of strength. Answer each question with a "**yes**" or "**no**."

	YES	NO
Can you do one chair stand (see page 26) without using your arms to assist you?		
Can you walk up and down a flight of 10 stairs without using the handrail to balance yourself?		
Can you stand unsupported on one foot for five seconds?		
Can you perform each of these exercises without discomfort?		

If you answered "no" to any of these questions, you can certainly still exercise, but you should do so in a supervised environment.

Designing your program

Before you lift even the lightest weight, you need to answer certain questions. How often should you work out? What are "reps" and "sets," and how many should you do? How much weight or resistance should you use? Why and for how long should you warm up, cool down, rest, and stretch? This section covers these issues and more. You will also learn what a well-rounded exercise program should include besides strength training (see "Current exercise recommendations," page 22). The workout calendar on page 25 should be helpful as you design your exercise program.

Frequently asked questions

Whether you're a beginner or more advanced, the answers to the following questions provide crucial information about strength training.

How often should I do strength training?

According to the most recent Physical Activity Guidelines for Americans, issued by the U.S. Department of Health and Human Services, adults ages 18 to 64 should perform a complete strength training routine two to three times a week. (Of course, once a week is better than not at all, if that's the most you can manage.) The fastest gains are made in the first four to eight weeks; after that, expect progress to slow somewhat.

How much rest do my muscles need?

Always allow at least 48 hours for muscles to recover between strength training workouts. So, if you do a full-body strength workout on Monday, wait until at least Wednesday to repeat it.

Some people prefer to break their strength training program into two components: upper body and lower body. In that case, you can perform upper-body exercises one day and lower-body exercises the next. Just make sure you work different groups of muscles on successive days, so your muscles can rest properly. And remember, you'll need to schedule at least two to three upper-body workouts and two to three lower-body workouts a week.

What are "reps" and "sets"?

Most strength training routines call for lifting and lowering a weight eight to 12 times, or repetitions ("reps"). That makes up one set. Typically, a complete workout includes two to four sets of approximately eight to 12 exercises that, combined, exercise all the major muscle groups.

What is good form?

One reason walking is such an easy type of exercise to recommend is that people already know how to do it. That's not true of strength training. Before you attempt a specific exercise, it's essential to learn the proper form, or technique, for the equipment and exercise you've chosen. Good form means aligning your body correctly and moving smoothly through an exercise. Focus on slow, smooth lifts and descents while isolating a muscle group. You isolate, or target, muscle groups by holding your body in a specific position while you contract or release certain muscles. As a result, you strengthen that targeted muscle group and avoid unnecessary strain on other muscles. In contrast, poor form can cause injuries and—at best—slow gains. (See "Training tips," page 24, for more on good form.)

Strength training machines help position you properly. But you still need to learn to adjust each machine to your body and use it correctly. If you're using free weights for resistance, good form is even more essential. Often, it helps to run through exercises the first few times without weights or with very little weight. A class or exercise professional can be instrumental in teaching good form. Videos—and to a lesser extent, books—can also help.

It's also a good idea to exercise in front of a mirror, at least initially. This allows you to observe your body position and to correct sloppy form.

How much weight or resistance should I use?

Once you understand exactly how to do each exercise, choose a weight that allows you to do only eight to 12 repetitions. The last one or two reps should be difficult. If you can't lift the weight at least eight times, use a lighter weight.

If you exercise regularly, your muscles will gradually adapt to the weight you are using so you can do more reps. When you can comfortably perform 12 reps without completely tiring the muscle, it's time to increase the amount of weight.

How many sets should I do?

Strength training focuses on tiring the muscles that are being worked. While some studies show you can net similar boosts in strength from performing just one set versus multiple sets, limited evidence suggests that two to four sets might be better. Multiple sets also have the edge when you first start training.

How long should I rest between sets?

If you don't rest at all, your muscles will be too tired to lift with good form. Resting for a minute between sets nets the best strength gains. Alternatively, cutting rest time between sets to 30 seconds keeps your heart rate up so you reap some aerobic benefits during a strength training session. It's wise to note, however, that this lessens strength gains. It's a tradeoff that each person should evaluate. If you do choose to cut your rest time, be sure you don't sacrifice good form.

Why should I warm up and cool down?

Any time you exercise, begin by warming up for five to 10 minutes, and end by cooling down for another five to 10 minutes. Warming up pumps nutrient-rich, oxygenated blood to your muscles as it raises your heart rate and breathing. Marching in place and gently swinging your arms or using a treadmill or exercise bike are all excellent ways to warm up. Start slowly, and gradually increase your pace. Unless a doctor or an exercise professional advises otherwise, aim for moderate exertion (see Table 2, at left).

Cooling down slows breathing and heartbeat, gradually routing blood back into its normal circulatory patterns. This helps prevent a sudden drop in blood pressure that causes dizziness, especially if you bend over or straighten up quickly (a reaction called postural hypotension). To cool down, gradually slow your movements or walk slowly until your heart rate and breathing are close to normal. Then do some stretching.

Why—and when—should I stretch?

Stretching can help you work kinks out of a stiff neck, ease back pain, and grasp a zipper that's been out of reach for years. Daily stretching gives you a greater range of motion and improves balance, too. Stretch after you've warmed up or at the end of a workout when muscles are warm and pliable.

Yoga, tai chi, and Pilates, which can be tailored to differing abilities and health concerns, combine stretching with relaxation. Studies show these activities enhance balance, lower blood pressure, and relieve stress, as well as improve flexibility.

Current exercise recommendations

Strength training, of course, is only one piece of the exercise puzzle. It's wise to keep the bigger picture in mind. A well-rounded program also includes aerobic activity, flexibility exercises, and balance exercises.

TABLE 2: How hard are you exercising?

EXERTION LEVEL	WHAT IT FEELS LIKE
At rest	No exertion
Very light	No noticeable exertion
Light	Noticeable exertion with breathing at a normal to slightly faster than usual rate
Moderate	Moderately vigorous exertion with deeper breathing, and with panting and sweating at the higher end of the range
Vigorous	Strong exertion with rapid breathing and heavy sweating
Very hard to extreme	Exercising at high intensity up to full capacity

▶ **A strong exercise routine**

For your exercise routine, aim for the following:

- at least 150 minutes of moderate aerobic activity, or 75 minutes of vigorous activity, or an equivalent mix per week (at least three sessions per week, with each session lasting at least 10 minutes)
- two to three sessions per week of strength training that exercises the major muscle groups of the legs, trunk, and arms and shoulders (or four to six weekly sessions if you plan to exercise only upper-body muscles on one day and lower-body muscles on the following day)
- balance exercises, either as part of your strength training routine or separately
- stretching exercises during the cool-down portion of each exercise session.

Aerobic activity (also called cardiovascular or endurance exercise), such as walking or swimming, speeds heart rate and breathing for sustained periods. According to the Physical Activity Guidelines for Americans, most adults should aim for at least 150 minutes of moderate aerobic activity per week or 75 minutes of vigorous activity—or an equivalent mix of the two. (Ten minutes of vigorous activity equals roughly 20 minutes of moderate activity.) Raising your weekly goal to five hours of moderate activity or two-and-a-half hours of vigorous activity nets additional health benefits. Spread your aerobic exercise across the week, if possible, so that you are performing it at least three days a week in episodes of at least 10 minutes each.

According to many exercise guidelines, running is an example of "vigorous" aerobic exercise. "Moderate" exercise might be walking at 4 miles per hour. The truth is, though, your level of fitness dictates whether an activity is light, moderate, or vigorous. If you are rarely active, a less-than-brisk walk might qualify as moderate—or even vigorous. Table 2 (page 22) can help you gauge your level of exertion. Many experts also offer the following rule of thumb for aerobic exercise: If you can talk easily while performing your routine, exercise harder. If you can't carry on a conversation at all, back off.

Flexibility exercises, or stretches, may expand your range of motion, keep muscles more limber, improve posture and balance, and help prevent falls. Warm muscles are less likely to be injured than cold muscles, so it's best to perform stretches as part of your cool-down following a workout. Or, if you prefer, you can stretch after a five- to 10-minute warm-up, during which you might walk or dance to some songs on the radio. Consider activities such as yoga or tai chi, which help with balance as well as flexibility. The American College of Sports Medicine recommends that older adults do flexibility exercises on the same days they do aerobic or strength activities, or at least twice a week.

Because regularly performing balance exercises can help protect against falls, it's wise to include these kinds of exercises in your routine. Here, you may be happy to note that your strength training routine can do double duty. Several of the strength training exercises described in this report also improve balance, particularly standing calf raises (page 26), chair stands (page 26), hip extensions (page 27), and side leg raises (page 32). In addition, we've included two additional balance exercises that are simple to perform (see "Balancing act," page 40).

A good exercise program builds slowly and safely on your current level of fitness. If you're a beginner, don't despair. Work up to these goals gradually. You'll find that some of these activities overlap nicely. For example, strength training has aerobic benefits if it raises your heart rate for sustained periods of time. You needn't follow a formula to know exactly how much faster than usual your heart should be beating—just pay attention to body signals that suggest you are exercising moderately (see Table 2, page 22). And remember to stretch as part of your cool-down.

Before you start: Schedules and training tips

Sometimes getting started is the toughest part of a new exercise program. Scheduling regular exercise sessions on a workout calendar (see sample on page 25) is a step on the right path. Marking progress monthly on the calendar can help keep you motivated.

Your workout calendar

Make copies of the blank calendar provided on page 25 and fill in the month and dates. Then decide what days and times work best for your strength training. Add in aerobic activities and flexibility exercises, too (see "Current exercise recommendations," page 22). Put a check mark on the days you exercise as intended. This can help you see when it's easiest to incorporate exercise into your schedule and where roadblocks tend to crop up. At the end of the month, review the calendar to see whether you need to make any adjustments in the timing of your workouts.

To help you get started, this section lays out two different strength training programs. Which one is the best match for you? If you aren't usually active, focus on the strength training program in Workout I (see page 26) and gradually add aerobic activities when you can. Even a few minutes a day will help, especially if you try to do a bit more week by week. Although it seems counterintuitive, strength training is a good way to build up muscles too weak for walking and other aerobic activities.

If you are in good shape, you may wish to use the strength training program in Workout II (see page 30), but be sure to include a few power training exercises from Workout I in your routine, too.

After you have completed one of these programs for 12 to 16 weeks, see the special section of this report ("Strength training over a lifetime," page 34), to find out how to maintain your strength gains and keep your strength training routine fun and challenging. ♥

Training Tips

These guidelines apply to any strength training program you may choose:

- Take five to 10 minutes to warm up before every session and cool down afterward; perform your cool-down until your breathing and heartbeat return to normal.

- Choose weights as light as 2 pounds for your first few strength training sessions so you can concentrate on good form. After that, add enough weight so that the maximum number of repetitions you can do per set is about eight to 12. The last few repetitions in each set should require a good deal of effort.

- Unless your doctor or an exercise professional gives you other instructions, lift weights to a three-second count. Pause for one second. Lower weights to a three-second count.

- Breathe out as you lift; breathe in as you lower. Don't hold your breath.

- Aim for two to three sets of eight to 12 repetitions each. When you are beginning a program, start with two sets of eight repetitions and work up from there; if you cannot perform eight repetitions initially, do as many as you can (or reduce the weight). When you can comfortably do two to three sets of 12 repetitions, increase the weight again. Muscles grow stronger only if you keep adding weight.

- Isolate muscles by trying to move only the muscles you're exercising. Don't rock or sway. Keep joints slightly bent rather than locked when you're extending the muscles.

- Rest between sets for a minute to reap the best strength gains.

- If you injure yourself, remember RICE (rest, ice, compression, and elevation). Rest the injured muscle. Ice it for 20 to 30 minutes every two to three hours during the first two or three days. Apply compression with an elastic bandage whenever you're out of bed until the swelling resolves. Elevate the injured area while resting or icing. Call your doctor for advice and information about managing pain or swelling. Wait until the injury heals before doing strength training on that muscle again, and start with a lower weight.

Workout calendar

Week: _____

SUNDAY	MONDAY	TUESDAY	WEDNESDAY	THURSDAY	FRIDAY	SATURDAY
Time:	Time:	Time:	Time:	Time:	Time:	Time:
Type of activity:	Type of activity:	Type of activity:	Type of activity:	Type of activity:	Type of activity:	Type of activity:
Time:	Time:	Time:	Time:	Time:	Time:	Time:
Type of activity:	Type of activity:	Type of activity:	Type of activity:	Type of activity:	Type of activity:	Type of activity:
Time:	Time:	Time:	Time:	Time:	Time:	Time:
Type of activity:	Type of activity:	Type of activity:	Type of activity:	Type of activity:	Type of activity:	Type of activity:
Time:	Time:	Time:	Time:	Time:	Time:	Time:
Type of activity:	Type of activity:	Type of activity:	Type of activity:	Type of activity:	Type of activity:	Type of activity:
Time:	Time:	Time:	Time:	Time:	Time:	Time:
Type of activity:	Type of activity:	Type of activity:	Type of activity:	Type of activity:	Type of activity:	Type of activity:
Time:	Time:	Time:	Time:	Time:	Time:	Time:
Type of activity:	Type of activity:	Type of activity:	Type of activity:	Type of activity:	Type of activity:	Type of activity:

Workout I: A strong beginning

Building the strength you need for daily tasks and recreation is one major goal of these exercises, which were designed with beginners of every age in mind. By focusing on muscles you actually use to walk up stairs, rise from a chair, or lift laundry or groceries, these exercises can help you regain lost abilities, if that's a problem for you. This is known as specificity—that is, choosing activities that target the specific muscles and moves needed for the tasks of daily life (or a sport) rather than just building up muscles in general.

The power moves described in this section can help you boost your ability to bring muscle force to bear quickly. That could make the difference between recovering from a misstep or falling after one.

Because this program has just nine exercises, it's easier to accomplish and less intimidating than many other strength training regimens. Focus on choosing challeng-

Workout I

1 Standing calf raise

Exercises the calf muscles

Stand with your feet flat on the floor. Hold on to the back of your chair for balance. Raise yourself up on the balls of your feet, as high as possible. Hold briefly, then lower yourself. Aim for eight to 12 repetitions. Rest and repeat the set.

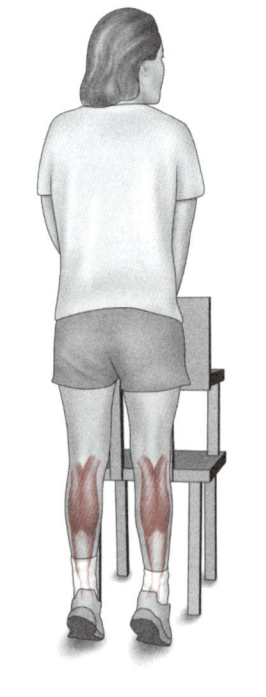

Variation: Once your balance and strength improve, tuck one foot behind the other calf before rising on the ball of your foot; do sets for each leg. Or stand on both feet, but do not hold on to a chair.

Power move: Change the move slightly for the final set by rising on the ball of your foot quickly. Hold briefly. Lower yourself at a normal pace.

2 Chair stand

Exercises the muscles of the abdomen, hips, front thighs, and buttocks

Place a small pillow at the back of your chair and position the chair so that the back of it is resting against a wall. Sit at the front of the chair, knees bent, feet flat on the floor and slightly apart. Lean back on the pillow in a half-reclining position with your arms crossed and your hands on your shoulders. Keeping your back and shoulders straight, raise your upper body forward until you are sitting upright. Stand up slowly, using your hands as little as possible. Slowly sit back down. Aim for eight to 12 repetitions. Rest and repeat the set.

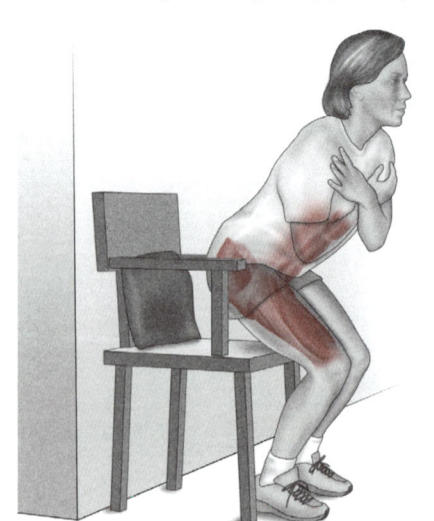

Power move: Change the move slightly for the last set by rising from the chair quickly. Sit down again at a normal pace.

ing weights and doing as much as you can. Remember, you must add to the weight you use whenever an exercise starts to feel easy (usually about every week or two).

Make it your goal to complete 12 to 16 weeks of Workout I, performing these exercises two to three times a week. If you do, you will notice many changes for the better. As you grow stronger, activities of all sorts will become easier. Simple tasks such as rising from a chair or going up stairs will no longer be a challenge. Sports may seem more enjoyable or simply become possible again. You may lose some weight or perhaps just feel as if you have, because your waistband will loosen as your abdominal muscles tighten. Even better are the changes you cannot see that put you on the road toward a healthier heart and bones and a lower risk of diabetes.

What you need. A sturdy chair (preferably with armrests), a small pillow, athletic shoes with nonskid soles, an exercise mat, and appropriate weights (see "Buying basic equipment," page 15) are all that you need for this simple workout.

The exercises

Before beginning the workout, complete a five- to 10-minute warm-up, such as walking briskly. As you perform each of these exercises, breathe out when you are lifting or pushing and breathe in as you release the muscle. Rest for one to two minutes between sets, and aim to complete two to three sets of each exercise.

Workout I

3 Stair climbing

Exercises the muscles of the front thighs and buttocks

Holding on to the handrail for balance if necessary, walk up and down a flight of at least 10 stairs at a pace that feels comfortable. Pause at the top only if you need to do so. Rest when you reach the bottom. Repeat four times.

Power move: If your balance is good, go up the stairs as briskly as you can and down at your normal pace for the last set.

4 Hip extension

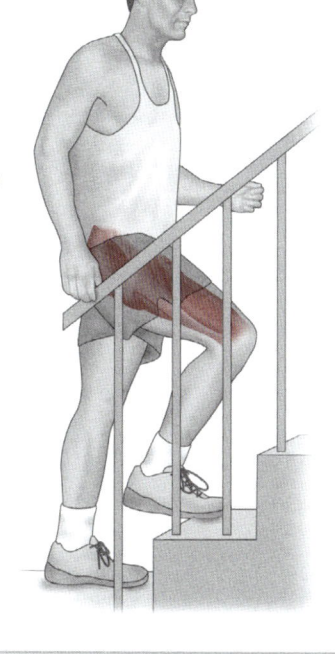

Exercises the muscles of the buttocks and back thighs

While wearing ankle weights, stand 12 inches behind a sturdy chair. Holding on to the back of the chair for balance, bend your trunk forward 45 degrees. Slowly raise your right leg straight out behind you. Lift it as high as possible without bending your knee. Pause. Slowly lower the leg. Aim for eight to 12 repetitions. Repeat with your left leg. Rest and repeat the sets.

Power move: Change the move slightly for the last set by rising from the chair quickly. Sit down again at a normal pace.

Workout I

5 Seated bridge

Exercises the muscles of the back thighs, back, and buttocks

Sit slightly forward in a chair with your hands on the armrests. Your feet should be flat on the floor and slightly apart, and your upper body should be upright (don't lean forward). Using your arms for balance only, slowly raise your buttocks off the chair until you are nearly standing, with your knees bent. Pause. Slowly sit back down. Aim for eight to 12 repetitions. Rest and repeat the set.

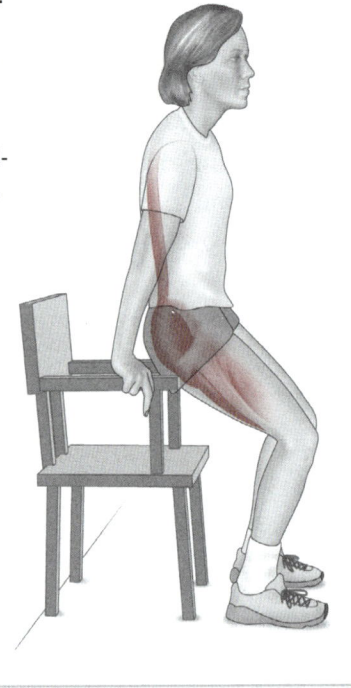

6 Biceps curl

Exercises the front upper arm muscles

Sit in a chair. Hold weights down at your sides with your palms inward. Slowly bend one elbow, lifting the weight toward your upper chest. As you lift, keep your elbow close to your side and rotate your palm so it faces your shoulder. Pause. Slowly lower your arm, rotating it back again so you finish with your palm facing your thighs. Aim for eight to 12 repetitions. Repeat with your other arm.
Rest and repeat the sets.

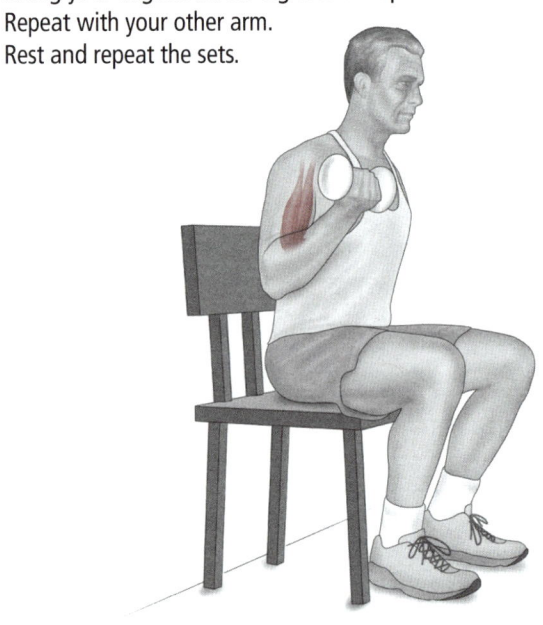

7 Triceps dip

Exercises the muscles of the back upper arms, chest, and shoulders

Put a chair with armrests up against a wall. Sit in the chair and put your feet together flat on the floor. Lean forward a bit while keeping your shoulders and back straight. Bend your elbows and place your hands on the armrests of the chair, so they are in line with your torso. Pressing downward on your hands, try to lift yourself up a few inches by straightening out your arms. Raise your upper body and thighs, but keep your feet in contact with the floor. Pause. Slowly release until you're sitting back down again. Aim for eight to 12 repetitions. Rest and repeat the set.

Variation: If you don't have a chair with armrests, sit on the stairs. Put your palms down on the stair above the one you are seated on. Press downward on the heels of your hands, lifting your body a few inches as you straighten your arms. Pause. Slowly release your body until you are sitting back down again. Aim for eight to 12 repetitions. Rest and repeat the set.

Power move: During your last set, lift your body quickly. Slowly release until you are seated again.

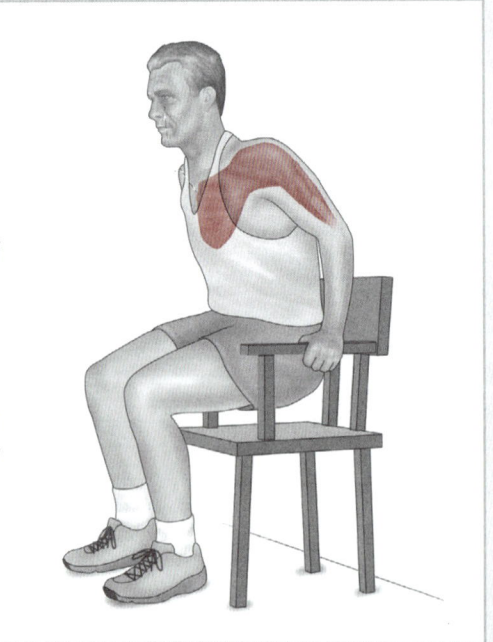

8 Curl-up*

Exercises the central abdominal muscles

Lie on your back on a mat. Put your hands beneath the small of your back and bend both knees to help stabilize your spine. Slowly raise your head and shoulders just a few inches off the floor. Pause. Slowly lower your head and shoulders. Aim for eight to 12 repetitions. Rest and repeat the set.

*If you have osteoporosis, talk to your doctor before trying this exercise. He or she may recommend that you avoid it.

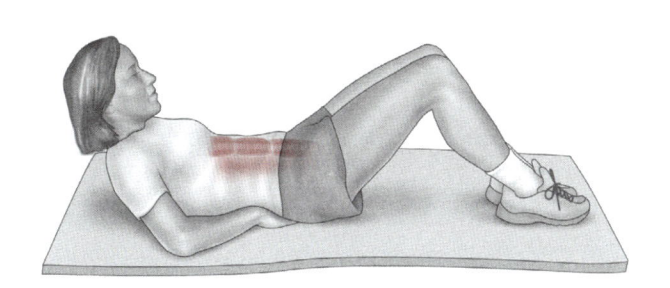

9 Standing side bridge

Exercises the lower back, side, and abdomen

Stand next to a wall, so the wall is on your right. Position yourself about two to three feet from the wall. Place your left foot directly in front of your right, and bend your right arm at your elbow. Lean your forearm against the wall so you are tilted toward it at about a 15-degree angle. Keep your body and spine in a straight line. (A) Hold that position for 30 seconds.

Now pivot on your toes, turning so you are facing the wall. Your feet should be side-by-side. Lean both forearms against the wall. Again, keep your spine straight; don't bend the torso. (B) Hold for 30 seconds.

Finally, pivot on your toes again so the wall is now on your left side. Your right foot should now be in front of your left, and you should lean against the wall on your left forearm. (C) Hold for 30 seconds. Rest, and repeat the whole sequence for another set. (While most exercises in this workout are performed eight to 12 times in a set, this exercise is only done once per set.)

Try to move from one position to the next as fluidly as possible, maintaining your spine in a straight line. Once you are comfortable with this exercise, increase the amount of time you hold each position by about 15-second increments, working your way up to two minutes at each step.

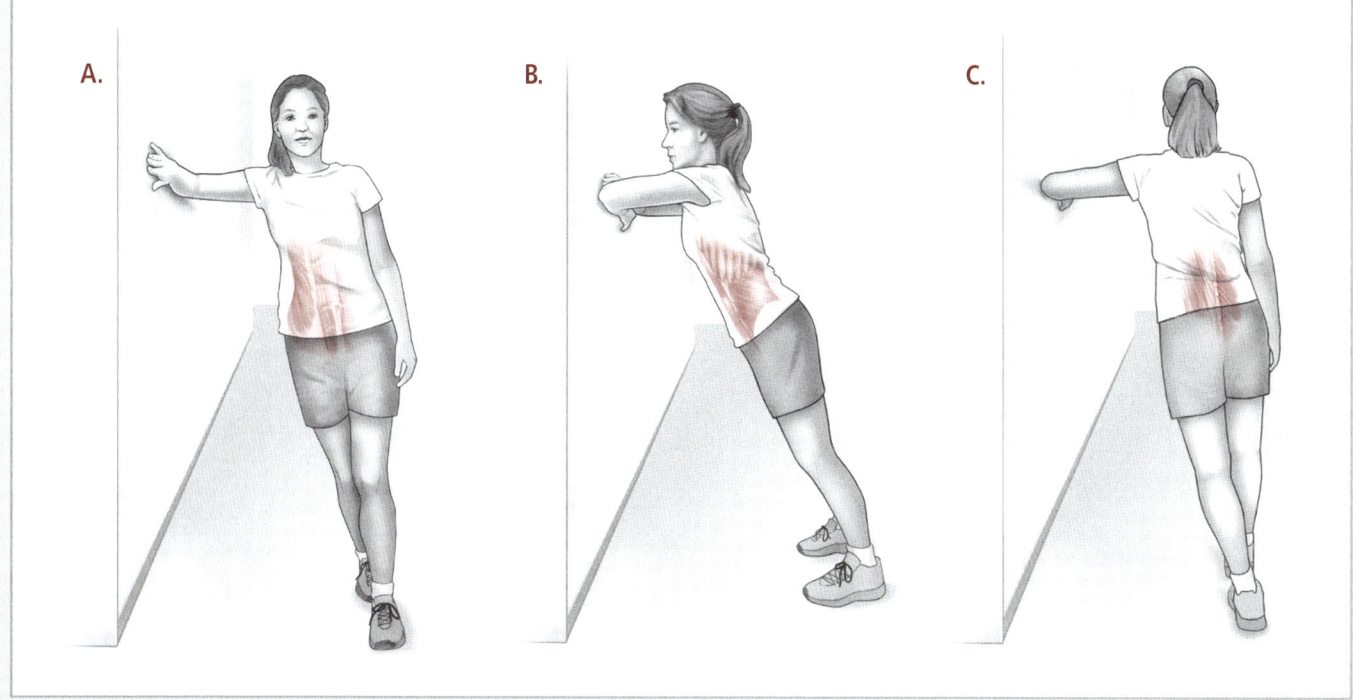

A.

B.

C.

Workout II: Stepping it up a notch

If you're reasonably active or have completed at least 12 to 16 weeks of Workout I, you may want more of a challenge. Workout II focuses on the same basic muscle groups, but offers several new exercises and variations on a few exercises from Workout I. It also calls for the same equipment as Workout I (with the possible addition of a weighted vest, if you want to turn this into a power workout; see "How to use a weighted vest," page 35).

Some people find changing their exercise program too daunting. If you feel this way, there's no need to switch from Workout I to Workout II. You can step up the Workout I program simply by adding weight, repetitions (up to a maximum of 12), and sets (up to a maximum of four), as appropriate (see "Stepping up the pace," page 34).

Workout II

1 Forward fly

Exercises the muscles of the shoulders and upper back

Sit in a chair holding weights about 12 inches in front of your chest. Your elbows should be up and slightly bent and palms should be facing each other (as if your arms are wrapped around a large beach ball). Lean forward at a slight angle in the chair, bending from your hips and keeping your back straight. Now, pull the weights apart while trying to bring your shoulder blades as close together as possible. Let the movement pull your elbows back as far as possible. Pause. Return to starting position. Do eight to 12 repetitions. Rest and repeat the set.

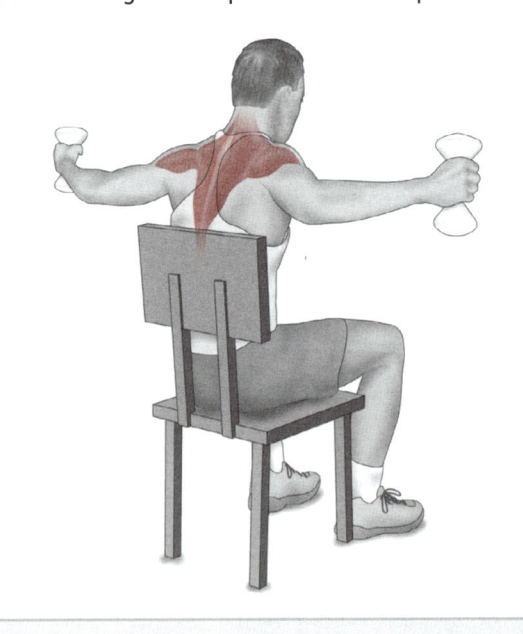

2 Overhead press

Exercises the muscles of the shoulders, upper back, sides of the rib cage, and back upper arms

Stand with your feet slightly apart. Hold a dumbbell in each hand at shoulder height (your elbows should be bent and the weights should be about six inches from your body). Hold the weights so your palms are facing forward. Slowly lift the weights straight up until your arms are fully extended. Pause. Slowly lower the dumbbells to shoulder level. Do eight to 12 repetitions. Rest and repeat the set.

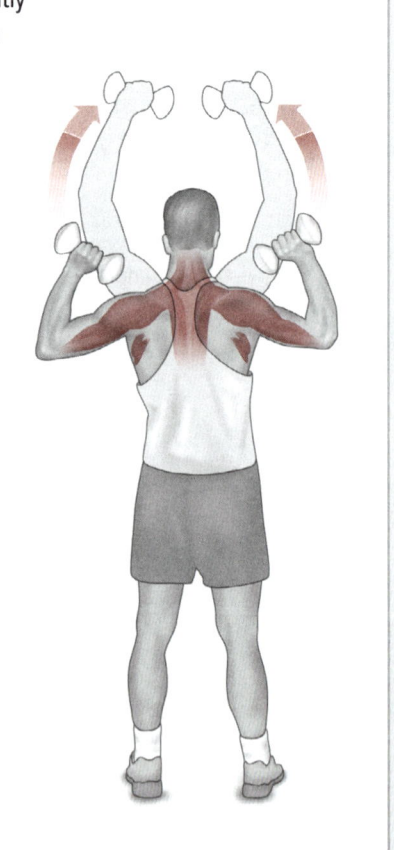

You'll see even more improvement, though, if you also add a few of the exercises from Workout II to your usual routine. Recommended additions are the forward fly, dumbbell squat, side leg raise, and back extension. Tacking on just one of these new exercises per week—or one every few weeks—may help you ease into a new routine.

The exercises

Do two to three sets of each of these 10 exercises. Don't forget to rest for one minute between sets for the best strength training gains. Make it your goal to complete 12 to 16 weeks of Workout II. Perform this strength training program two to three times each week. Remember to avoid holding your breath as you exercise. Breathe out when you're lifting or pushing and breathe in as you relax the muscle. You must keep challenging yourself as the routine becomes easier if you wish to continue to reap gains.

In addition to the exercises in this section, continue to do the four power moves described in Workout I (explained in the standing calf raise, chair stand, stair climbing, and triceps dip descriptions). If doing just one set seems too easy, try two or three. Or, if you prefer, you can turn up the power by wearing a weighted vest for those four exercises.

Workout II

3 Triceps extension

Exercises the back upper arm muscles

Begin by standing with your feet slightly apart, holding weights with your palms facing behind you. Lift the weights straight up. As you lift, you'll be raising your elbows up and bending them at about a 90-degree angle. Your shoulders should not hunch up and your elbows should not be any higher than your shoulders. If you feel any shoulder pain, lower your arms slightly. This is the starting position. While keeping your elbows at the same level, slowly raise your lower arms so that your arms are outstretched. Pause. Slowly return to the starting position. Do eight to 12 repetitions. Rest and repeat the set.

Variation: An alternative to this exercise is the triceps dip in Workout I (see page 28).

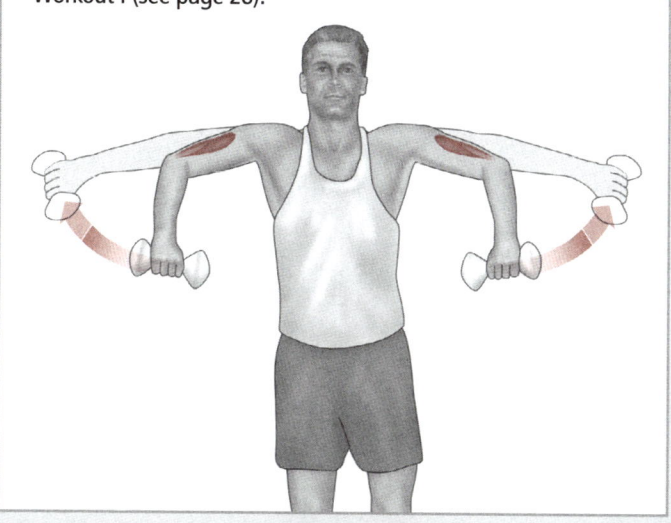

4 Double biceps curl

Exercises the front upper arm muscles

Stand or sit holding dumbbells down at your sides with your palms facing inward. Slowly bend both elbows, lifting the weights toward your upper chest. Keep your elbows close to your sides. As you lift, rotate your palms so they face your shoulders. Pause. Slowly lower your arms to the starting position. Do eight to 12 repetitions. Rest and repeat the set.

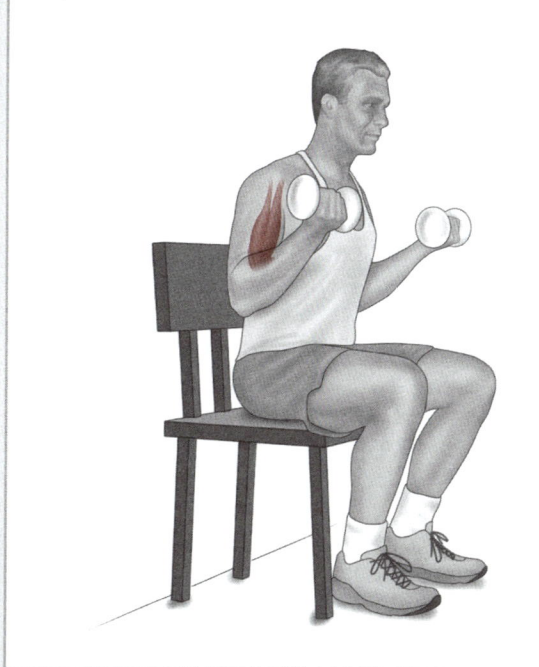

Workout II

5 Dumbbell squat

Exercises the muscles of the buttocks and front thighs

Stand with your feet shoulder-width apart. Hold a weight in each hand with your arms at your sides and palms facing inward. Slowly bend your knees, lowering your buttocks about eight inches while continuing to hold the weights at your sides. Keep your back in a neutral position or very slightly arched as you do this. Pause. Slowly rise to an upright position. Do eight to 12 repetitions. Rest and repeat the set.

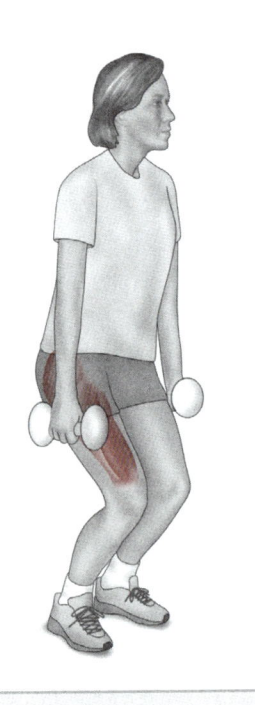

6 Side leg raise

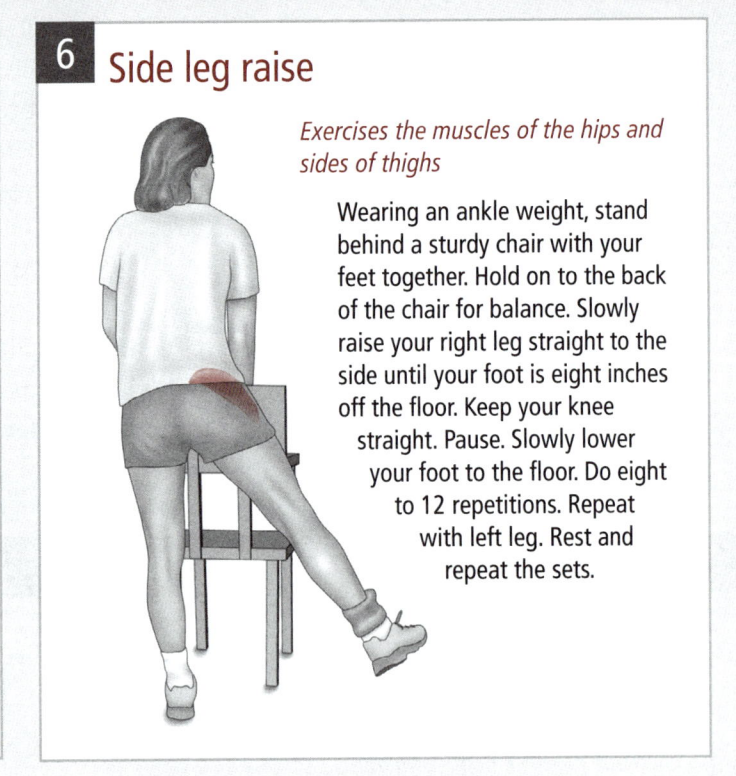

Exercises the muscles of the hips and sides of thighs

Wearing an ankle weight, stand behind a sturdy chair with your feet together. Hold on to the back of the chair for balance. Slowly raise your right leg straight to the side until your foot is eight inches off the floor. Keep your knee straight. Pause. Slowly lower your foot to the floor. Do eight to 12 repetitions. Repeat with left leg. Rest and repeat the sets.

7 Bridge

Exercises the muscles of the back, back thighs, and buttocks

Lie on your back on a mat with your knees bent and your feet flat on the floor. Put your hands next to your hips with palms flat on the floor. Keep your back straight as you lift your buttocks as high as you can off the mat, using your hands for balance only. Pause. Lower your buttocks without touching the mat, then lift again. Do eight to 12 repetitions. Rest and repeat the set.

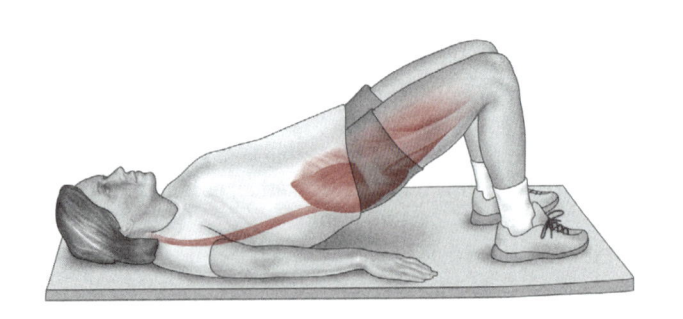

8 Advanced curl-up

Exercises the abdominal muscles

Lie on your back on a mat. Put your hands beneath the small of your back and bend both knees to help stabilize your spine. While contracting your abdominal wall muscles so your navel is pulled toward your spine, raise your head and shoulders a few inches off the floor. Pause. Lower your head and shoulders. Do eight to 12 repetitions. Rest and repeat the set.

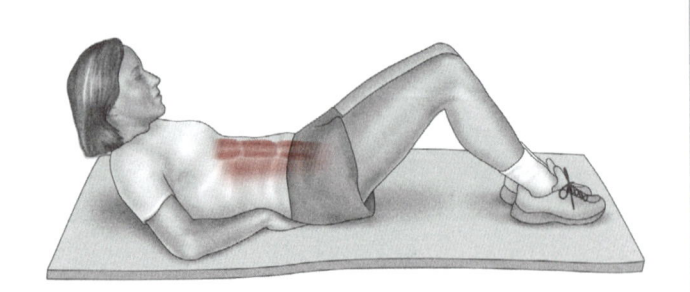

Workout II

9 Side bridge

Exercises the muscles of the lower back and abdomen

Lie in a straight line on your left side on a mat. Bend both knees at a 90-degree angle so that your calves and feet point behind you. Raise your upper body, supporting it on the side of your left forearm. (Your left elbow should be bent at a 90-degree angle directly below your shoulder, and your forearm should point forward.) Now you are in the starting position. Slowly lift both hips a few inches upward to create a bridge until only your left forearm, knee, calf, and foot are touching the mat. Your spine should be in a neutral position (so it's in a straight line and isn't curved or arched). Pause. Lower yourself to the starting position. Do eight to 12 repetitions. Repeat on your right side. Rest and repeat the set.

Advanced move: Assume the starting position, but keep your legs straight. You can put your right leg behind your left leg to steady yourself, if you like. Once you are ready, slowly lift both hips a few inches upward to create a bridge until only your left forearm and foot are touching the mat. Pause. Lower yourself to the starting position. Do eight to 12 repetitions. Repeat on your right side. Rest and repeat the set.

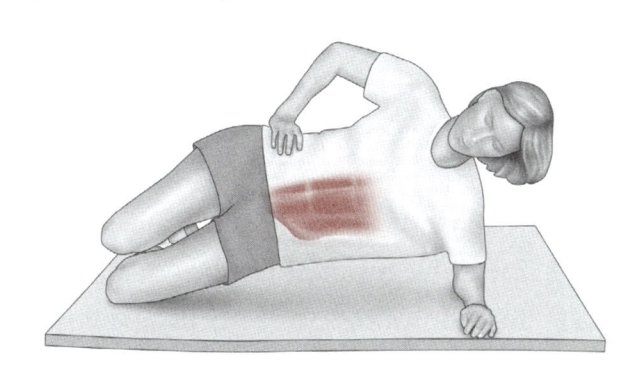

10 Back extension

Exercises the muscles of the back, hips, and buttocks

Find a sturdy counter that reaches about waist level. Face it, standing a couple of feet away. Distance yourself so that when you lean against the counter your body is at about a 30- to 45-degree angle. Keeping your body straight and your arms across your chest (as if you are hugging yourself), lean forward so that you are resting your weight against the counter. Hold for one minute. Rest and repeat for another set. (While most exercises in this workout are performed eight to 12 times in a set, this exercise is only done once per set.)

Advanced move: If you wish to push yourself further, you can work up to holding this position for two minutes, rather than one. Or instead of keeping your arms crossed during the move, reach your right arm up above your head so it is in a straight line with your torso and extend your left leg backward, raising it just an inch or two off the floor. Hold for 30 to 45 seconds. Then alternate your arm and leg (lift your left arm and extend your right leg).

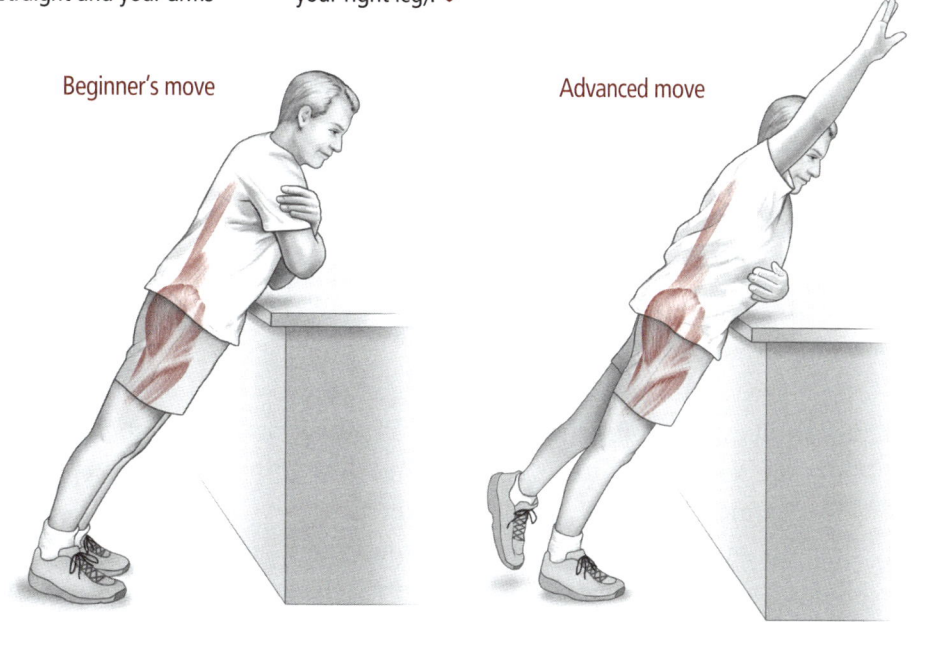

Beginner's move

Advanced move

www.health.harvard.edu

Strength and Power Training 33

SPECIAL SECTION

Strength training over a lifetime: Keys to staying motivated

Measurable progress can be one of the biggest motivators for success with any behavior change, whether you are trying to lose weight, exercise more often, or quit smoking. The satisfaction you derive from seeing how your new behaviors have begun to affect your health—or your waist size—can entice you to keep going even if you are growing tired of the same old routine. However, in order to make strength training a lifelong endeavor, it's a good idea to vary your routine and crank up the degree of challenge so you keep it fun and fresh.

Charting your progress

Probably the best way to keep track of your progress is to test yourself over time. Do so before you start an exercise program and then repeat the tests monthly, recording your results in the accompanying chart (page 36). This written record can provide encouragement and help you stay motivated, because you'll see steady improvement if you stick to an exercise program.

The National Institute on Aging recommends testing not only strength, but also endurance, lower-body power, and balance. Because strength training affects all of these—and a well-rounded exercise plan addresses the full quartet—the tests suggested in the chart should provide a good snapshot of your progress.

The chart has space for you to write down a few personal goals: Why do you wish to do strength training? Are you hoping to tone your muscles? Boost energy? Or simply muster the strength to heft your own groceries or walk easily up a flight or two of stairs? Jotting down positive changes that you notice each month can help keep you exercising.

How soon can you expect to see gains? Research suggests the biggest gains occur within the first four to eight weeks of strength training. After that, you should still progress, but most likely at a slower pace.

This chart covers six months. If you copy the blank chart, you can continue testing yourself after that, too. Write in the name of the month, the results of the tests, and changes you've observed in your abilities. Try to check your progress on the same day of each month and at the same time of day, if possible.

Stepping up the pace

Because your body adapts to whatever demands you regularly place upon it, you must gradually make your workout more difficult to continue improving your fitness. This can also keep you challenged and interested in your fitness routine.

You are ready to increase the challenge whenever your current regimen becomes too easy to accomplish. There are several ways to do this:

■ **Add repetitions.** Aim for the maximum of 12 repetitions; after that, increase weight.

■ **Add a set.** Perform three or four sets of each exercise instead of

Strength and Power Training   www.health.harvard.edu

Strength training over a lifetime | **SPECIAL SECTION**

How to use a weighted vest

If you want to wear a weighted vest when doing the power moves described in this report, choose one that can hold a total of 20 to 40 pounds in half-pound bars. The maximum amount of weight you use in your vest depends on your body weight. The chart on the right can help you determine the upper limit that's right for you.

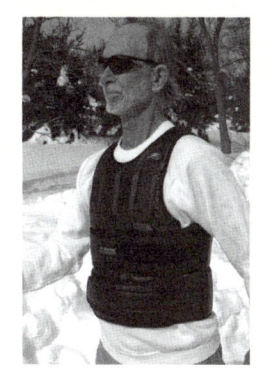

Begin by wearing the vest without any weights. After two to three workouts with just the vest, add weight in the amount described in the chart. Increase the weights in your vest every week or two, in the same increments. Once the total reaches the upper limit set for your body weight, stop adding weights.

For example, a 120-pound woman would add 2 pounds to her vest every week or two. Over the course of about six to 12 weeks, the weight in her vest would increase as follows: the vest alone, 2 pounds, 4 pounds, 6 pounds, 8 pounds, 10 pounds, and finally 12 pounds. She should not put more than 12 pounds into her vest.

Guidelines for adding weight to your vest

If you weigh:	Increase the weight in your vest at regular intervals by this amount	Maximum amount to use in your vest
75–99 pounds	1 pound	7 pounds
100–149 pounds	2 pounds	12 pounds
150–199 pounds	3 pounds	18 pounds
200–239 pounds	4 pounds	20 pounds
240–280 pounds	5 pounds	25 pounds
281–329 pounds	6 pounds	30 pounds
330 pounds or more	7 pounds	35 pounds

If your workout feels too vigorous at any time or if you can't complete the recommended two to three sets of an exercise with the vest on, reduce the amount of weight in your vest to a more comfortable level.

Photo courtesy of Ironwear Fitness

---

two. After that, increase the weight or change another parameter, such as repetitions or exercises.

■ **Add weight.** This is an easy change to make—up to a point. If you're using ankle weights for lower-body work, you may need to do additional exercises to make further gains, or you might need to switch to machines, which will allow you to use heavier leg weights (more than 20 pounds). When you add weight, drop back to two sets if you have been doing three or four, until that seems too easy. For power training, you can also try a weighted vest (see "How to use a weighted vest," above).

■ **Add exercises.** If you are performing Workout I, you may want to add a few exercises from Workout II. If you are already doing Workout II, you can add some exercises from "Switching up your routine" on page 38.

Keeping it interesting

If you feel yourself balking at the thought of one more day of the same old routine or find you've reached a plateau, consider making some changes. The following suggestions can help you add variety to your workout.

■ **Mix it up.** Vary your program by switching the order in which you do the exercises. Although committed bodybuilders deliberately move in sequence from larger muscles to smaller muscles, the rest of us needn't follow such an absolute order.

■ **Try new equipment.** Substitute one type of equipment for another if you belong to a gym that offers a good range. For example, try working out with machines instead of free weights one day a week or switching from one brand of machine to another. Alternately, you might try exercises using a medicine ball, resistance bands, or resistance tubing. A good trainer can help.

www.health.harvard.edu

Strength and Power Training

SPECIAL SECTION | Strength training over a lifetime

Progress chart

ACTIVITY	1ST MONTH	2ND MONTH	3RD MONTH	4TH MONTH	5TH MONTH	6TH MONTH
Strength: Biceps curl (see page 28) Write down the weight lifted and number of sets of biceps curls you are able to do.	Weight: Sets:	Weight: Sets:	Weight: Sets:	Weight: Sets:	Weight: Sets:	Weight: Sets:
Strength: Chair stand (see page 26) Time how long it takes to do 10 chair stands. Aim to do chair stands without using your arms to help. If you needed to use your arms, circle "arms"; otherwise, circle "no arms." Be sure to exercise at a safe pace.	Time: Arms No arms	Time: Arms No arms	TTime: Arms No arms	Time: Arms No arms	Time: Arms No arms	Time: Arms No arms
Lower-body power Time yourself as you go briskly up a flight of at least 10 stairs, then walk down it at your usual pace. If that seems way too easy from the start, try going up and down the stairs two or three times. Use the same stairs and number of trips each time.	Time:	Time:	Time:	Time:	Time:	Time:
Balance Time how long you can stand unsupported on one foot. Do this on each foot for as long as you can.	Left: Right:	Left: Right:	Left: Right:	Left: Right:	Left: Right:	Left: Right:
Endurance Time how long it takes you to walk four blocks or 400 yards. Use the same course each time.	Time:	Time:	Time:	Time:	Time:	Time:
Personal goals 1. 2. 3. 4.	Changes	Changes	Changes	Changes	Changes	Changes

Strength and Power Training

www.health.harvard.edu

- **Make substitutions.** You can swap exercises that focus on strengthening the same basic muscle groups. That is, choose a different exercise that works leg muscles or upper arm muscles. You can use the examples found in "Switching up your routine" on page 38 or get ideas from other publications on strength training, as well as exercise videos and classes.
- **Change your pace.** Vary the intensity of your workouts. For example, do one hard, one medium, and one lighter workout in cycles of seven to 10 days. This is a form of periodization—an exercise strategy that can enhance strength gains, help sidestep boredom and plateaus, and avoid overtraining while allowing more time for the body to heal after being thoroughly taxed. Reps, sets, and resistance for different exercises are varied to achieve these goals. Because it can be difficult to put together a good periodization strategy, it's essential to work with an exercise professional to come up with a plan that's right for you.
- **Work out with a friend when you can.** If your friend is careful about good form, too, this can be a way to help reinforce good habits. Some gyms have a buddy board to help members find workout partners.
- **Join a six-week or three-month class.** The camaraderie and supervision can be helpful, plus you'll probably learn something new.
- **Work with a trainer.** Pay for a session or two with a certified personal trainer who can help you develop a well-rounded new routine.
- **Put on music that raises your spirits.** Some people even find it possible to exercise to a favorite TV show. While that generally works best with aerobic exercises that require little thought, you may find it is appropriate for strength training, too.

Maintaining gains

Muscles stay strong with regular workouts, but the gains slip away quickly if those workouts stop. To keep building strength and power and to achieve the fullest gains possible, continue strength training for two to three days a week.

At some point, though, you may wish to step down to a strength training maintenance program. Your goals can help guide you in determining whether to make this change. Engaging in strength training twice a week offers the best assurance that you'll be able to hold on to the gains you've made in all your muscle groups. If you're very busy, though, some evidence suggests that training once a week can preserve strength—at least for certain muscles.

One study showed that older men who had done three sets of knee extension exercises three times a week for 12 weeks exhibited no loss in strength when workouts were cut to once a week. Meanwhile, a control group lost significant size and strength in muscles after ceasing activity entirely. Similar findings from other studies bolster this. Still, most experts recommend aiming for two weekly sessions instead of one.

If you do decide to cut back to one day a week of strength training during a vacation or for a longer period of time, replace it with other activities. This can help you stay in good shape and lead a healthy, active, and independent life.

SPECIAL SECTION | Strength training over a lifetime

Switching up your routine

You can freshen up a stale routine by substituting exercises that target the same basic muscles. Here are a few options to pick and choose from.

Thigh raise

Exercises the muscles of the hips and front thighs

Wearing ankle weights, stand with your hands on your hips. Raise one foot, keeping a toe on the floor. Keeping your back straight, raise your knee up until your thigh is parallel to the floor (your foot will be lifted off the floor). Pause. Lower the leg to the starting position. Do eight to 12 repetitions. Repeat with the opposite leg. This is one complete set. Rest and repeat the set.
Variation: Stand next to a chair and hold on to the back of it for balance, if necessary. Raise the knee that's farthest away from the chair up toward your chest. Pause. Lower the leg. Do eight to 12 repetitions. Rest and repeat the set. Then move to the other side of the chair and repeat with your other leg.

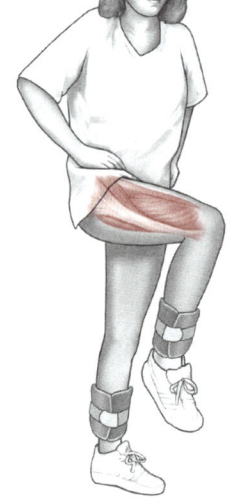

Knee flexor

Exercises the back thigh muscles

Wearing ankle weights, stand behind a chair with your hands on the back of it. Bend one knee to bring your foot close to the back of your thigh, keeping your back straight and your upper leg as still as possible. Pause. Lower leg to starting position and repeat with opposite leg. Do eight to 12 repetitions. Rest and repeat the set.

Knee squeeze

Exercises the inner thigh muscles

On a mat, lie on your back with your knees bent and your feet flat on the floor. Place a ball about the size of a soccer ball between your knees. Squeeze your thighs together as hard as you can for a count of three. Release and repeat. Do eight to 12 repetitions. Rest and repeat the set. (Alternatively, you can do this exercise standing. Simply place the ball between your knees and squeeze hard for three seconds.)

Push-up

Exercises the muscles of the chest and back upper arms

Hold your body straight above a mat with your palms flat on the mat at shoulder level and your elbows slightly bent. Only your toes and palms should be touching the mat. Your feet may be together or a bit apart. Keeping your back as flat as possible, bend your elbows more to bring your trunk several inches closer to the floor without allowing your trunk to hit the mat. Then push yourself back upward until your arms are extended, without locking your elbows. Return to the original position and repeat. Aim for eight to 12 repetitions. Rest and repeat the set.

Variations: If a full push-up is too challenging, try knee push-ups, balancing your weight on your knees instead of your toes. Or do wall push-ups. Stand up straight in front of a wall with your arms extended at shoulder height. Put your palms against the wall with the fingers pointing upward. Bend your elbows to lower your upper body as far as possible toward the wall, keeping a straight line from head to heel. Pause, then push away from the wall to return to the starting position, maintaining neutral alignment from head to toe throughout the movement. Do eight to 12 repetitions. Rest and repeat the set.

Strength training over a lifetime | **SPECIAL SECTION**

Horizontal stabilization (also known as "bird dog')

Exercises the muscles of the buttocks, spine, and shoulders

On a mat, get down on your hands and knees. Look down at the floor, keeping your neck straight. Inhale as you slowly extend your right leg and left arm. Keep your back flat while doing this. Pause. Exhale as you return to the starting position. Do eight to 12 repetitions. Repeat with your left leg and right arm. Rest and repeat the set.

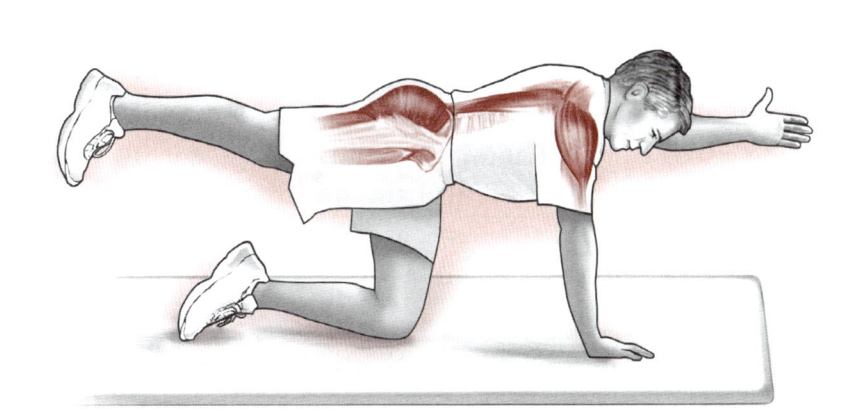

Upright row

Exercises the muscles of the shoulders, upper back, and front upper arms

Stand with your feet shoulder-width apart. With your arms at your sides, hold a dumbbell in each hand. Your palms should be facing your thighs. Slowly lift both dumbbells straight up your sides to shoulder height. As you lift, keep the weights close together and close to the front of your body by pointing your elbows outward. Pause. Slowly lower the dumbbells back down to your thighs. Do eight to 12 repetitions. Rest and repeat the set.

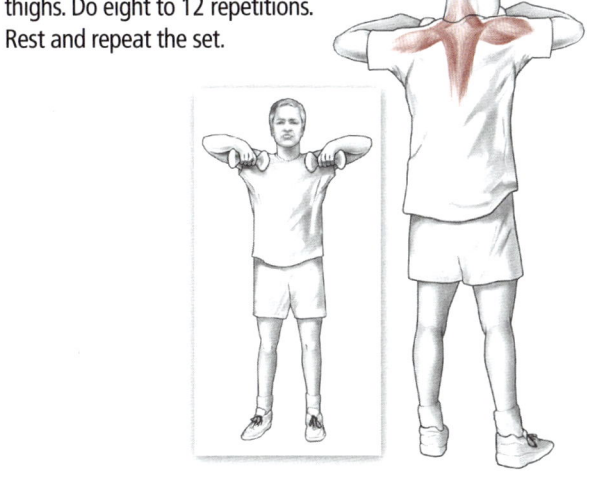

Trends in training

Incorporating new gear can spice up your exercise routine

Variety adds spice to all parts of life, and working out is no different. Equipment like medicine balls, resistance bands and tubes, kettle bells, and the Bosu have grown in popularity because they can add challenge and interest to your routine.

The three strengthening tools below can prevent you from becoming complacent or bored. Talk with a personal trainer about whether they're right for you.

- **Medicine balls** are used for core and strength exercises and are available in a variety of weights. They are about the size of a soccer ball.
- **Resistance bands** look like big, wide rubber bands and come in several levels of resistance, designated by color.
- **Resistance tubing** comes in several levels of resistance, also coded by color. Look for tubing with padded handles on each end. Some brands come with a doorknob attachment helpful for anchoring the tubing in place when doing certain exercises. ▼

www.health.harvard.edu

Strength and Power Training

Balancing and stretching exercises

A complete exercise program should also include some balance and flexibility exercises. Adding these into your routine needn't be difficult or time-consuming. As you'll see, your current routine may already include some balance-improving exercises. Stretching is also an important, if frequently overlooked, part of a routine. Note that the stretches shown in this section can also serve as your cool-down after strength training or aerobic activity.

Balancing act

Several of the strength training exercises provided in Workout I and Workout II also help improve balance. So if you're regularly performing exercises such as the standing calf raise (page 26), chair stand (page 26), hip extension (page 27), and side leg raise (page 32), you may already be doing all you need to keep yourself steady on your feet. But if you aren't performing these exercises regularly or if you would like to further enhance your

Stretching exercises

1 Calf stretch

Stretches the Achilles' tendon and calf

Stand in front of a wall. Stretch out your arms so that your palms are flat against the wall and your elbows are almost straight. Keeping your right knee slightly bent, step back a foot or two with your left leg, positioning the heel and foot flat on the floor. Hold for 30 seconds. Now bend your left knee while still keeping the heel and foot flat on the floor. You should feel these stretches in your calf and Achilles' tendon; if you don't feel a stretch, move your foot back a bit farther. Hold for 30 seconds. Switch legs and repeat.

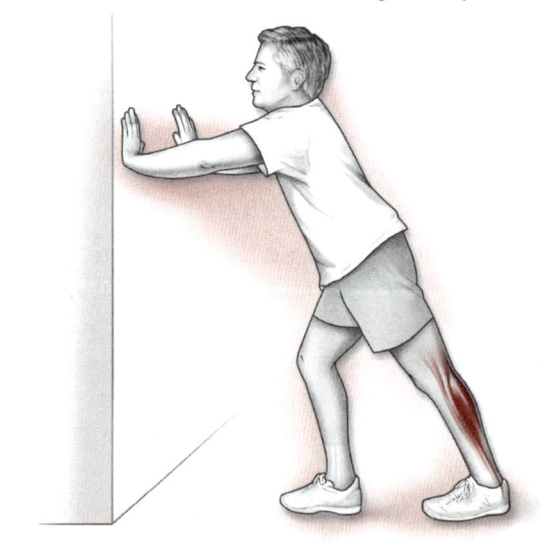

2 Thigh stretch

Stretches the front of the thigh

Stand next to a wall so you can touch it for balance if necessary. Keeping one leg straight, bend your other knee and grasp your ankle to pull your heel up toward your buttock. Hold for 30 seconds. Switch legs and repeat.

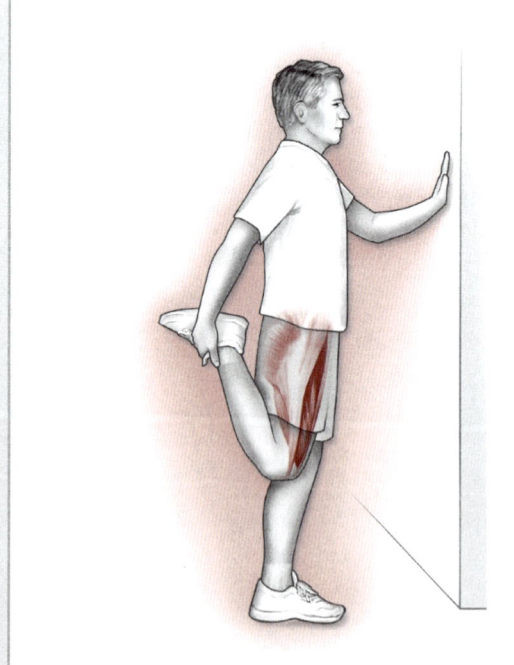

balance, you may want to try the following two exercises. These exercises can be done anytime—every day of the week or just a few times a week.

Heel-to-toe walk

Position your heel just in front of the toes of the opposite foot each time you take a step. Heel and toes should actually touch as you walk forward for eight to 12 steps. If necessary, steady yourself by putting one hand on a counter as you walk at first, and then work toward doing this without support. Repeat two to four times.

Single leg stance

Stand on one foot for up to 30 seconds. Put your foot down and rebalance yourself, then repeat on the opposite leg. Perform two to four times on each leg. If this is too difficult, you can steady yourself by holding on to the back of a chair or a counter at first. Then work toward doing this without support.

Stretching

Experts disagree about whether stretching prevents injury, mainly because there is a lack of hard evidence to this effect. We do know, however, that shorter, stiffer muscle fibers, which are an unfortunate result of getting older, may make you vulnerable to injuries. This can happen either because bones and joints are more easily pulled out of alignment, or simply because a tight muscle is more likely to

Stretching exercises

3 Hamstring stretch

Stretches the back of the thigh

Stand far enough behind a chair that you can hold the back of it with both hands and also bend over at your hips until your torso is parallel to the floor. Try to keep your back and shoulders straight so that you feel the stretch in the back of your thighs. Hold the position for 30 seconds.

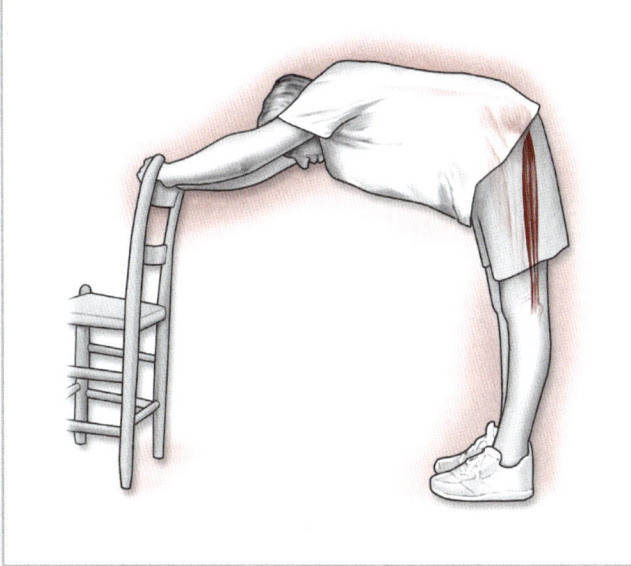

4 Double hip rotation*

Stretches the back and hips

Lie on your back with your knees bent and feet flat on the floor. Keep your shoulders on the floor throughout the exercise. Gently lower both legs to one side, keeping your knees together, and turn your head to the opposite side. You should feel this stretch along the muscles of your hip, side, and, to a lesser extent, neck. Hold for 30 seconds. Bring your knees back to center and repeat on the other side.

*If you have had a hip replacement, talk to your doctor before trying this stretch. He or she may recommend that you avoid it.

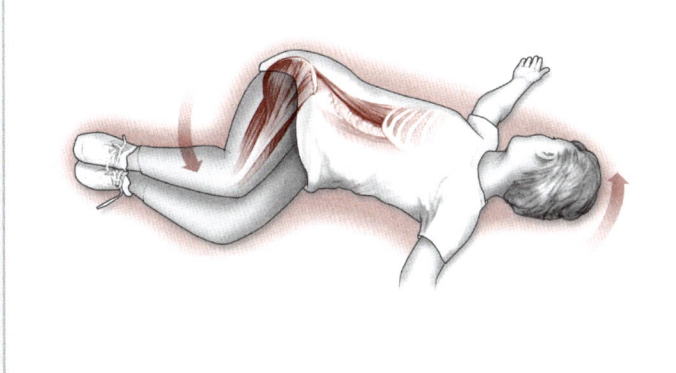

tear under stress than one that is more flexible. We also know that when done correctly, stretching helps loosen tight muscles, keeping you more limber. It also gives you a greater, more comfortable range of motion and improves posture and balance.

So, regardless of whether there is proof that stretching actually prevents injury, it is an important part of overall musculoskeletal health. Experts used to recommend stretching before exercising, but newer research suggests that the best time to stretch is after exercising, as part of your cool-down session, because that is when muscles are most pliable. Stretching during your workout is fine, too, and may help boost flexibility, according to a small study on lower-leg and ankle stretching sponsored by the American College of Sports Medicine.

Some stretches to try

Once your muscles are warmed up, you can do these

Stretching exercises

5 Hip flexor stretch

Stretches the hip

Stand facing a chair, with the back of the chair against a wall for support. Raise your left foot up and rest it flat on the chair, with your knee bent. (Or you may prefer to place your foot on a stairstep, so that you can hold the railing for balance.) Keeping your spine as neutral as possible, press your pelvis forward gently until you feel a stretch at the top of the right thigh. Your pelvis will move forward only a little; the movement is subtle. Hold for 30 seconds. Repeat on the other side.

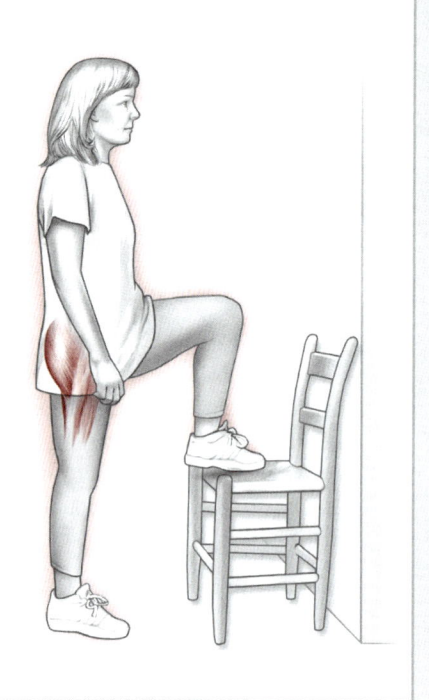

6 Side stretch

Stretches the side, shoulder, and arm

Stand or sit up in a chair. Reach upward with your right hand as far as you can while letting your left hand slide gently downward. You should feel this stretch along your rib cage, trunk, and waist. Hold for 30 seconds. Switch sides and repeat.

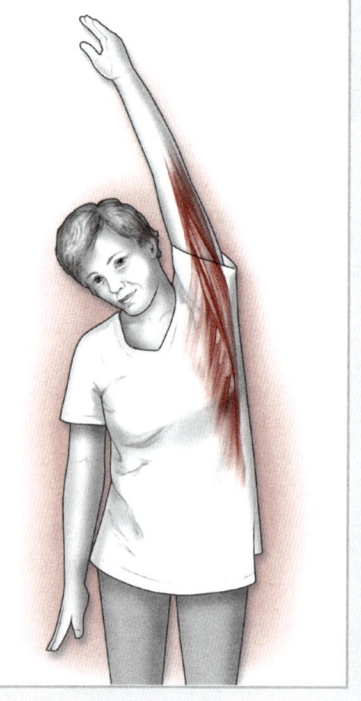

7 Shoulder rotation

Stretches the upper back, upper chest, and shoulders

Lie on your back on a mat with a pillow under your head. Stretch your legs out straight, or put a rolled towel beneath your knees if that's more comfortable. Extend your arms straight out to the sides, then bend your elbows so your hands point to the ceiling. Your shoulders and upper arms should remain flat on the mat. Now slowly roll your arms back toward the mat, stopping when you feel a stretch in your shoulders. Hold for 30 seconds. Raise your arms slowly until your hands are pointing back at the ceiling. Roll your bent arms forward toward the floor. Again stop when you feel a stretch in your shoulders. Hold for 30 seconds.

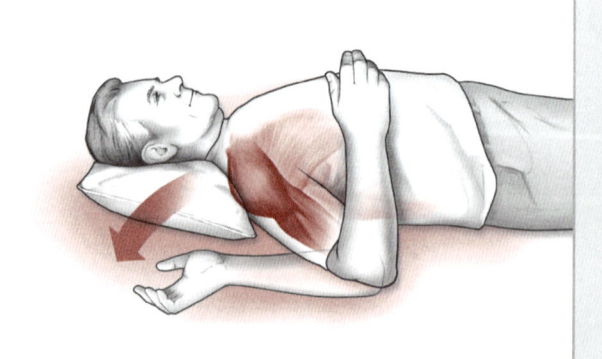

stretches anytime during the course of your workout. Some people like to do a stretch or two after each exercise; others prefer to stretch as part of their cooldown. Whichever you choose, be sure to hold each stretch for 10 to 30 seconds and repeat it three or four times. If you hold the position for less time or do fewer repetitions, you won't lengthen the muscle fibers as effectively. On the other hand, holding a stretch for too long can increase your chances of injuring the muscle. When you are starting out, you may find that it's useful to time your stretches. Breathe normally, and don't bounce or overextend your body so that a stretch hurts. Stop immediately if you feel sharp pain.

If you have had a joint replaced or repaired, ask your surgeon whether you need to avoid certain stretches, such as the double hip rotation. If you have osteoporosis, consult your doctor before doing floor stretches or stretches that bend the spine. ▼

Stretching exercises

8 Hip and lower back stretch

Stretches the hips and lower back

Lie flat on your back with both legs extended. Keep your neck on the floor, but look down toward your chest. Bend both knees and clasp them with your hands, pulling your knees toward your shoulders as far as they will comfortably go. Breathe in deeply and exhale, bringing the knees closer as you breathe out. You will feel compression in your hips and a stretch in your lower back. Hold for 30 seconds while breathing normally.

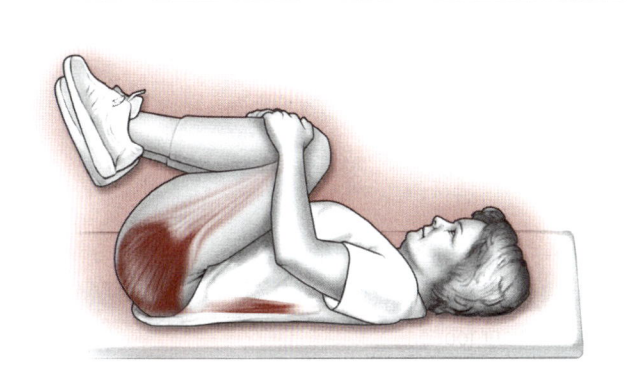

9 Inner leg stretch

Stretches the inner thigh

Sit on a mat with your knees bent and pointing outward, and your feet together. Draw your feet close to your body. Holding your shins or feet with your hands, bend your upper body forward and press your knees down with your elbows. Hold for 30 seconds.

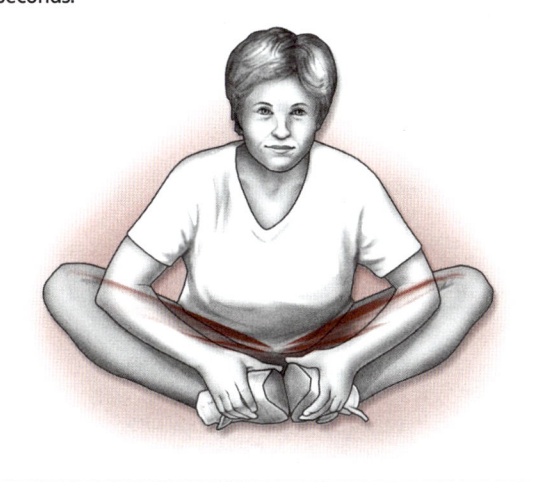

10 Triceps stretch

Stretches the triceps, rotator cuff, and upper back

Bend your right arm behind your neck, pointing your elbow toward the ceiling. Grasp your elbow with your left hand. Pull the raised right elbow gently toward the left until you feel a mild stretch at the back of your right upper arm. Hold for 30 seconds. Repeat with left arm.

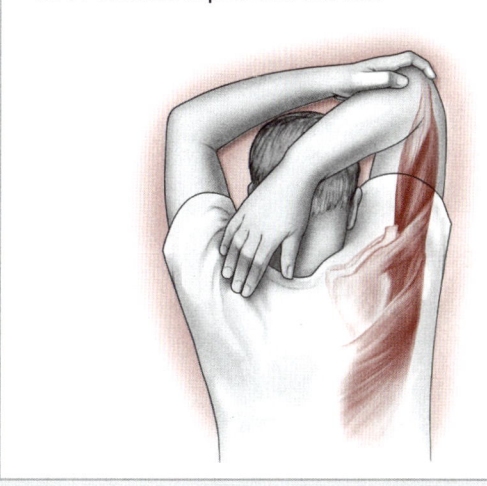

Resources

Publications

Better Balance: Easy exercises to improve stability and prevent falls
Suzanne Salamon, M.D., and Brad Manor, Ph.D., Medical Editors
With Josie Gardiner and Joy Prouty, Master Trainers
(Harvard Medical School, 2012)

In young, healthy adults, balance is largely an automatic reflex. However, gradual changes linked to growing older—such as weak or inflexible muscles, slower reflexes, and worsening eyesight—can erode your sense of balance. For this Harvard Special Health Report, two physicians with expertise in balance and aging team join forces with two master trainers to develop safe, effective exercises to help prevent falls, build better awareness of your body, boost your confidence, and keep you healthy and independent. Order online at www.health.harvard.edu or call 877-649-9457 (toll-free).

Core Exercises: 6 workouts to tighten your abs, strengthen your back, and improve balance
Edward M. Phillips, M.D.
With Josie Gardiner and Joy Prouty, Master Trainers
(Harvard Medical School, 2011)

Want to bring more power to pursuits like swimming, golf, and tennis? Ward off or ease lower back pain? Build up your balance and stability so that you're less likely to fall? A strong, flexible core underpins all these goals. When you're ready to take your training up a notch, this Special Health Report is a logical next step. Order online at www.health.harvard.edu or call 877-649-9457 (toll-free).

Exercise in Rehabilitation Medicine
Walter Frontera, M.D., David M. Dawson, M.D., and David Slovik, M.D.
(Human Kinetics, 2006)

Edited by three Harvard Medical School experts, including one of the original medical editors of this report, this textbook offers an in-depth look at exercise, including explanations of how exercise affects muscles and body systems and the role of exercise in treating a wide variety of illnesses.

The No Sweat Exercise Plan: Lose Weight, Get Healthy, and Live Longer
Harvey Simon, M.D.
(McGraw-Hill, 2006)

Written by a Harvard doctor, this book gives a unique point of view on the "light" exercise most people do every day, be it cleaning the house or walking the dog. The book features the No Sweat Exercise Pyramids—a set of practical, visual guides that show the types and amounts of exercise required for good health.

Organizations

American Academy of Physical Medicine and Rehabilitation
9700 W. Bryn Mawr Ave., Suite 200
Rosemont, IL 60018
847-737-6000
www.aapmr.org

This national organization is for doctors who specialize in physical medicine and rehabilitation for musculoskeletal and neurological problems. AAPMR offers referrals to these doctors and information on a variety of conditions such as low back and neck pain, spinal cord and brain injuries, osteoporosis, and arthritis.

American College of Sports Medicine
401 W. Michigan St.
Indianapolis, IN 46206
317-637-9200
www.acsm.org

This nonprofit organization is devoted to expanding scientific knowledge about exercise and developing programs for health and exercise professionals. ACSM offers several types of certification in sports medicine, health, and fitness for health and exercise professionals as well as information on strength training and other forms of exercise for the general public.

American Council on Exercise
4851 Paramount Drive
San Diego, CA 92123
888-825-3636 (toll-free)
www.acefitness.org

This nonprofit organization promotes fitness and a healthy lifestyle. ACE certifies fitness professionals and also offers educational materials and consumer information on finding and evaluating a personal trainer.

American Physical Therapy Association
1111 N. Fairfax St.
Alexandria, VA 22314
800-999-2782 (toll-free)
www.apta.org

This national professional organization fosters advances in education, research, and the practice of physical therapy. The website has a search engine to help locate board-certified clinical specialists who have additional training in specific areas of physical therapy.

Arthritis Foundation
1330 Peachtree St., Suite 100
Atlanta, GA 30309
800-283-7800 (toll-free)
www.arthritis.org

This nonprofit organization offers free publications on many arthritic conditions as well as information on exercise, research, and current treatments.

National Institute on Aging
Building 31, Room 5C27
31 Center Drive, MSC 2292
Bethesda, MD 20892
800-222-2225 (toll-free)
www.nia.nih.gov

This government agency, part of the National Institutes of Health, offers free health and fitness publications for older adults, including exercise guides in English and Spanish and a DVD on exercise.